Contact Information

(210) 859-6573

admin@ChristFitFusion.com

www.ChristFitFusion.FIT

www.facebook.com/ChristFitFusion

www.ChrisitFitFusion.wordpress.com

Register of Copyrights, United States of America. Copyright Registration Number: TXu 1-898-024
Effective date of registration: January 4, 2014

Index

It's FREE! And ANY "BODY" can do it! Whether you're young, old, out of shape, disabled or have six toes. It doesn't matter. Fitness is for you and just like salvation, it's Free. It's also very simple and doesn't require a lot of fancy equipment or expensive memberships. But just like Christianity it gets too complicated. Although the message is "simple" the follow through is one of the hardest, most challenging yet Rewarding things you'll ever do. The journey is full of trials, tribulations, pain (both good and bad), perseverance, successes, failures, plateaus, growth, and letting go of some selfish pleasures, but ultimately it leads to Victory! Are we talking about salvation or fitness here? You tell me. It applies to both.

Christ Fit is the fusion of spiritual and physical fitness. It is built on three key principles; 1. Eat a healthy spiritual and physical diet. 2. Exercise spiritually and physically. 3. Do them both consistently. **Simple. Challenging. Effective.** Live the right lifestyle and the results will take care of themselves. God put Christ Fit in my heart several years ago. I have a passion and a gift for fitness and I do genuinely care about helping you get healthier and into better shape, but I care equally if not more about your spiritual fitness than I do about your physical. Christ Fit combines the two. I find so many parallels in the quest to become and stay physically fit and the quest for spiritual fitness. I have spent over 20 years in the fitness industry and have been pursuing my spiritual hard body for almost 15 years (Still a long way to go). Christ Fit is the out flow of some of what I have learned along the way and also what God has revealed to me. I by no means claim to have all the answers or abide by everything in this journal flawlessly. I struggle to get it right every day and during the writing of Christ Fit I felt as much like I was preaching to myself as anybody else.

Why do Christ Fit? Why journal? Because keeping a journal works. It's been proven over and over again. Those who journal what they put into their bodies lose more weight even when not on a "diet" than those who are on a "diet," but don't record their nutritional intake. If you journal what you eat you will become fitter. You have to take action and write it down though. It's kind of like reading your Bible. God gave us His Word. It's got everything we need to know in order to follow Jesus and live a Christian lifestyle. It's got all the answers. If we read it and obey it our lives change. But we have to read it and **obey it**. There has to be the follow through. You have to see a need for change, want to change and you have to participate in the process. Nothing will work unless you are committed and take action.

Journaling is such a great tool for fitness. I used to do it "religiously" in my own training. Not only did I record every single thing that I ate or drank including the number of calories, grams of protein, carbohydrates, and fats, but I also recorded every single workout that I did. My workout partner and I would record how many repetitions and how much weight we used for every set of every exercise we did in the gym.

Journaling gives you such Awareness. It allows you to keep track of successes and failures so you can effectively chart the right course and make adjustments when necessary. It helps you detect patterns and identify where your strengths and weaknesses are.

Journaling is nothing new. Athletes, coaches, dieticians and trainers have done it for decades. Most every professional diet and nutrition "program" advertised on TV these days use some form of journaling. It works. Aren't we as Christians, spiritual athletes? Aren't we as Christians supposed to take care of our physical bodies as well? Christ Fit is the fusion of spiritual and physical fitness. Take your fitness seriously; both your spiritual and physical fitness. If journaling works for helping you lose fat and get in shape, I propose that it will help you lose spiritual fat and get into better spiritual shape as well.

• A 2006 Purdue study found that fundamental Christians are by far the heaviest of all religious groups led by the Baptists with a 30% obesity rate compared with Jews at 1%, Buddhists and Hindus at 0.7%

• A 2011 Northwestern University study tracking 3,433 men and women for 18 years found that young adults who attend church or a Bible study once a week are 50% more likely to be obese than those who do not attend.

• The Pawtucket Health Program found that people who attended church were more likely than non-church members to be 20% overweight and have higher cholesterol and blood pressure numbers.

• A 2001 Pulpit and Pew study of 2,500 clergy found that 76% were overweight or obese compared to 61% of the general population at the time of the study.

Stoll, M.D., Scott. "Fat in Church." FoxNews.com. 4 Jan. 2013. Web.

The following is my suggestion on how to use the Christ Fit journal. First of all read the entire journal from front to back (pay particular attention to day 31). Christ Fit didn't all come in one night, but that's where the bulk of it started. I really felt God prompting me to sit up in bed one night at about 2 a.m. and start writing down some things as they relate to physical fitness and their analogies with spiritual fitness. So I did. I didn't know where it was going, but I wrote it all down and then over time it got segmented up into separate pages for a thought of the day format.

I'd like you to read the entire journal first and here's why. Every individual page of the journal makes sense in and of itself but I want you to have the big picture going into the first day so that there is no confusion or misunderstandings along the way. It's kind of like if you turned to Matthew 5:48 and read "But be perfect, even as your Father in heaven is perfect," and then turned to Philippians 1:5 and read "And I am sure that God, who began the good work within you, will continue his work until it is finally finished on that day when Christ Jesus comes back again." Well how in the world am I expected to be perfect if I am a work in progress? It might be a little confusing and even seem contradictory if you didn't know the whole context. Christ Fit is by no means of biblical stature, but there could likewise be some seemingly contradictory material if you don't have the full perspective. And it's not like I'm asking you to read the entire Bible first. It's only a few Christ Fit pages, c'mon.

My second suggestion is that when you do get started that you be brutally honest. Write down everything; the good, the bad, and the ugly. The journal entries are broken down into 4 quadrants: Spiritual Diet, Physical Diet, Spiritual Exercise, and Physical Exercise. There are some sample journal entries to show you how to record them. Basically spiritual exercise is action and spiritual diet is what you consume spiritually. Examples of spiritual exercise are things like reading your Bible, an action and a discipline (Coincidentally what you read is also spiritual nutrition and you could list it in your spiritual diet section as well). Other examples of spiritual exercises are prayer, fasting, choosing to listen to a teaching on your way to work, sharing your faith, forgiving someone, etc.

Spiritual diet is just like our physical diet. It's what we consume: Read I Corinthians 13 about love, listened to a sermon on heaven by Chip Ingram on the way to work, listened to praise and worship music during lunch, watched a raunchy movie/read Cosmo after dinner (Yes, there is spiritual junk food)... Write it down.

With physical exercise I suggest that you record as much detail as possible, but here's the deal. It will be easy to write down such things like: 30 minute aerobics class, walked around neighborhood for 20 minutes, did 5 sets of 5 push-ups with 1 minute in between, did 2 sets of 25 crunches, got up out of recliner and walked to the fridge 3 times... But for those of you who are working out at home or end up in the gym doing multiple sets of multiple exercises I have included an additional training journal page for you to record the details of your workouts and help you chart your progress. It's not hard to find yourself eventually doing 20 to 30 total sets throughout the course of a workout when you're really into a strength training program. Good luck trying to remember all the details from day to day. Use it if you need it and then all you have to do in the Christ Fit journal that is split up into fourths, is write down "30 minutes of weight training," "30 minute circuit-training class," or whatever the case may be. If you decide that it's a tool you want to use then feel free to make yourself copies and do so. Don't get overwhelmed. At the very least just record a simple entry of what you did for physical exercise on the multi section journal page that accompanies each day's topic.

In regards to your physical diet I suggest writing down the time you eat, what you eat, and the quantity of what you eat. Again, don't get overwhelmed. In the beginning keep it simple if you need to. Just write down a description like "1 palm sized grilled chicken breast," "1 cup green beans," "1/2 cup brown rice," etc. As you progress you can get more detailed with actual calorie counts, and grams of protein, carbohydrates, and fats. That's what the additional Christ Fit Diet Journal is for. If you find yourself using the more detailed diet journal page there is no reason to record it as well on the first multi section journal page. Right now just get in the routine of making good choices, writing it down, and using your God given common sense. Don't over complicate anything in the beginning. You have to crawl before you can walk. Like the more detailed training journal, if you find that you want to use the more detailed nutrition journal then make yourself copies from the blank one you will find with the samples and use it.

Thirdly, take your journal with you as much as possible. There's no way you're going to remember everything at the end of the day. Journal as you go.

Lastly, use the notes section to write down anything that you want or need to. Maybe something that convicted you in the reading that day or a thought that you need to focus on and affirm throughout the day. Write down reminders and goals for yourself as you mentally plan your Christ Fit strategy for the day. Record benchmarks, successes, where you're struggling or need extra focus.

Above all, use it. If you miss a day then don't sweat it. Pick up where you left off, but really try to develop the habit of journaling every day.

I'm sure that you're going to have many questions as you work through this Christ Fit journal. It is written so that you will have questions but not because I don't want to answer them. Many of your questions will have many good answers and I want to avoid claiming to have "the" answer as so many other fitness professionals do to promote their product or nutrition plan. I have no problem answering questions and walking with you through your Christ Fit journey. I will be your coach, mentor, trainer, guide or whatever you need, but I will also push you to educate yourself and workout your own salvation so to speak. If you can make it to a Christ Fit class then it would be great to visit with you in person. If you want to host a Christ Fit class at your church or with a group of friends, contact us and we will make that happen. At the very least you can reach me at www.facebook.com/ChristFitFusion or www.ChristFitFusion.FIT and I will be happy to answer your questions.

Some Christ Fit Scriptures

Let me say first of all that Christ Fit is a Christ centered approach to spiritual and physical fitness. It does not however, contain a lot of "christianeze." I use analogies and perspectives to connect our spiritual and physical fitness and they are all inspired by scripture and biblical truth. I just don't write with a lot of preachy lingo. The following scriptures are provided as a reference to give you an idea of where my thoughts are coming from and how God has used them to inspire the Christ Fit message and journal. They are in no particular order in relation to the flow of the journal, but you will find all of them throughout the process of working through it.
All scriptures are new living translation unless other wise noted.

MATTHEW 6:33: (New King James Version) But seek first the kingdom of God and his righteousness, and all these things will be added to you.

If you're living the right lifestyle the results will take care of themselves.

ROMANS 12:1-2: And so dear brothers and sisters, I plead with you to give your bodies to God. Let them be a living holy sacrifice – the kind he will accept. When you think of what he has done for you, is this too much to ask? Don't copy the behavior and customs of this world, but let God transform you into a new person by changing the way you think. Then you will know what God wants you to do, and you will know how good and pleasing and perfect his will really is.

We've heard for years that the divorce rates and various other struggles within the church are comparable to those of the world. It is no different with our physical fitness and eating habits either; especially if you're a pot-lucking Baptist. But it seems easy to apply this scripture to things like sexual promiscuity and other "important" moral issues. Why is it not on the spiritual radar that our behavior and customs should be "set apart" here as well? Not that we can't enjoy a good potluck or a desert now and then, but why does it seem like we treat our gluttony, obesity and general poor health like it's not a real sin? There's nothing like hearing a good sermon on self-control and abstaining from harmful substances from an unhealthy preacher with a food addiction. Shouldn't we let God transform our thinking in the area of our eating and exercise as well? Our physical condition as Christians is as much of a disgrace when compared to the world as is our divorce rate, promiscuity, and other behaviors.

II CORINTHIANS 10:4-5: We use God's mighty weapons, not mere worldly weapons, to knock down the Devil's strongholds. With these weapons we break down every proud argument that keeps people from knowing God. With these weapons we conquer their rebellious ideas, and we teach them to obey Christ.

There are many weapons that our enemy can use against us and he knows just which ones we are susceptible to and can do us the most harm and hold us back from being all God has planned for us. Even something as simple as our physical condition can have an impact on our psyche and cause us to feel defeated and not worth much which can lead to apathy in regards to our spiritual condition as well. It also works the other way around. Many people eat as a coping mechanism due to various moral and spiritual failures and struggles. Either way, we have God's weapons to knock down strongholds. Take hold of the fact that you are a creation of God, important to Him, and His dwelling place. We're in a fight. When in a fight you both strike and get hit. We have access to God's armor, but we have to choose to use it.

GALATIANS 6:7-9: Don't be misled. Remember that you can't ignore God and get away with it. You will always reap what you sow! Those who live only to satisfy their own sinful desires will harvest the consequences of decay and death. But those who live to please the Spirit will harvest everlasting life from the Spirit. So don't get tired of doing what is good. Don't get discouraged and give up, for we will reap a harvest of blessings at the appropriate time.

The message of reaping what we sow is as straight forward a message as they come. Whether positive or negative, you name it and there's a consequence for it. Plant good seed and reap a healthy harvest. Plant weeds and well… you know. Whether spiritually or physically we reap what we sow and we are the sewers responsible for what kind of seed we are planting. Take care of your garden. I get it that life gets tiring at times. Don't give up. The rewards and the harvest are worth the perseverance.

JOSHUA 24:15: But if you are unwilling to serve the Lord, then choose today whom you will serve. Would you prefer the gods your ancestors served beyond the Euphrates? Or will it be the gods of the Amorites in whose land you now live? But as for me and my family, we will serve the Lord.

We all serve something and inevitably our allegiance is often divided. Serving God is a choice. How we serve Him is a choice. We're all called to serve and obey Him and many times the personal, private areas of obedience are the hardest, but choose whom you will serve. Either get on board or get off. Whatever you choose do it whole heartedly. It is your choice to be Christ Fit or not.

EPHESIANS 4:11-14: He is the one who gave these gifts to the church: the apostles, the prophets, the evangelists, and the pastors and teachers. Their responsibility is to equip God's people to do his work and build up the church, the body of Christ, until we come to such unity in our faith and knowledge of God's Son that we will be mature and full grown in the Lord, measuring up to the full stature of Christ. Then we will no longer be like children, forever changing our minds about what we believe because someone has told us something different or because someone has cleverly lied to us and made the lie sound like the truth.

The devil tells us many lies: "You're not special;" "Your spouse isn't into you;" " '_____' will make you happy;" "All you need is '_____' to succeed;" "This pill makes fat scientifically 'melt' off;" "You're not good enough;" "You'll never be in shape." Fitness, both spiritual and physical, is often laced with lies. Not every time, but many. Many times the truth is stretched or the message is glamorized so that it will sell. Don't believe the lies! The problem is that many lies can sound like the truth when you don't have a solid foundation and when you aren't seeking the truth for yourself. It's not that you can't trust anyone, but unless you are seeking the truth for yourself and developing discernment you are susceptible to being misled and taken advantage of for the gain of someone else. There are no short cuts and there are no miracle solutions that do it for you. Discipline yourself, educate yourself, feed on a healthy spiritual and physical diet and grow up mature and full grown in the Lord so that you will not buy into the lies.

MATTHEW 5:48: But be perfect, even as your Father in heaven is perfect.

Well, there's the standard. We are called to be perfect. We all know we're not, but we should certainly strive for it with a healthy dose of reality.

I THESSALONIANS 5:17-18: Keep on praying. No matter what happens, always be thankful, for this is God's will for you who belong to Christ Jesus.

Pray without ceasing. Never stop praying. What if it said eat without ceasing or never stop eating. Maybe then this would be one scripture that some would take literally. Let's put this in perspective. We are to stay in an ever present mind set of prayer. We don't drive around or sit at our desks with our heads bowed and hands folded all the time. But it is possible to keep God in our thoughts and mental conversations at all times. It's also possible to feed on little bits of his word throughout the day without having to keep your nose buried in the Bible.

We aren't called to "gorge" on God's word or pray 24 hours a day but we are essentially told to "graze" on it. Our bodies of course work so much better when we graze on food rather than gorge once or twice a day. Not on pizza and sugar of course, but when we have a steady consumption in small doses of healthy nutrition (spiritually and physically) our spirit and bodies naturally speed up their metabolism, crave more of the good stuff and get healthier and fitter.

EPHESIANS 5:18: Don't be drunk with wine, because that will ruin your life. Instead, let the Holy Spirit fill and control you.

We are instructed to pray continuously, throughout our day every day and to be continuously filled (literally be being filled) with the spirit. A little prayer at dinner or before bed isn't enough. A warm fuzzy feeling at church once in a while isn't enough. We need a steady flow every day and it isn't that difficult to do. Implement a little prayer and worship music or teaching on the way to work; maybe even something playing at your desk. Do the same thing on the way home. I like to keep scripture cards on my desk. You get the idea. It's the same thing with our diet and exercise. You've heard of the grazing approach to eating. Just like these scriptures address prayer and being filled with the spirit, we should have a consistent flow of nutrition throughout our day, not just one or two meals. And don't fill your body or spirit with crap. Be continuously filled with spiritual and physical nutrition. The more you fill up on healthy stuff the less you will crave the unhealthy. So eat without ceasing. Just make sure it's healthy and in proper portion.

MATTHEW 10:32-33: If anyone acknowledges me publicly here on earth, I will openly acknowledge that person before my Father in heaven. But if anyone denies me here on earth, I will deny that person before my Father in heaven.

Acknowledge Jesus. Let the cat out of the bag. Be bold. Be proud. Don't be afraid to tell others. Tell someone about your fitness commitment too. It's good for positive pressure and accountability.

PHILIPPIANS 1:6: And I am sure that God, who began the good work within you, will continue his work until it is finally finished on that day when Christ Jesus comes back again.

While perfection is our calling and our goal, we are truly a work in progress. As we strive to become more Christ Fit we must focus on our progress not perfection. Failures are not fun and we shouldn't treat them flippantly, but we must also look at the big picture. As long as we are moving in the right direction and can identify progress we can know that we are in the process of becoming more Christ Fit.

PHILIPPIANS 3:12-14: **I don't mean to say that I have already achieved these things or that I have already reached perfection! But I keep working toward that day when I will finally be all that Christ Jesus saved me for and wants me to be. No, dear brothers and sisters, I am still not all I should be, but I am focusing all my energies on this one thing: Forgetting the past and looking forward to what lies ahead, I strain to reach the end of the race and receive the prize for which God, through Christ Jesus, is calling us up to heaven.**

However you've blown it in the past, whether you've blown your diet, done the walk of shame back home, or failed to let go of a grudge… However you've gotten off track you can have a change of heart, repent, draw a line in the sand and move forward. Keep your eye on the prize and get back in the race!

EPHESIANS 6:10-13: **A final word: Be strong with the Lord's mighty power. Put on all of God's armor so that you will be able to stand firm against all strategies and tricks of the Devil. For we are not fighting against people made of flesh and blood, but against the evil rulers and authorities of the unseen world, against those mighty powers of darkness who rule this world, and against wicked spirits in the heavenly realms. Use every piece of God's armor to resist the enemy in the time of evil, so that after the battle you will still be standing firm.**

We are in a fight and we need to realize it. God has given us access to His armor, but we have to choose to put it on. I can't imagine a soldier going into battle without his armor on, but that is what we do every day when we enter into the day without our spiritual armor. Armor can be heavy and battles can be grueling. Both require strength. We're in a battle and we must become Christ Fit to survive it.

I CORINTHIANS 9:24-27: **Remember that in a race everyone runs, but only one person gets the prize. You also must run in such a way that you will win. All athletes practice strict self-control. They do it to win a prize that will fade away, but we do it for an eternal prize. So I run straight to the goal with purpose in every step. I am not like a boxer who misses his punches. I discipline my body like an athlete, training it to do what it should. Otherwise, I fear that after preaching to others I myself might be disqualified.**

Go all in. Run with purpose. Run to win. We are spiritual athletes. That requires discipline and self-control. Run straight to the goal. Don't take any unnecessary steps. Make a plan both in your spiritual and physical fitness. Make a plan, be committed to it, and be deliberate in how you execute it.

II TIMOTHY 4:7: **I have fought a good fight, I have finished the race, and I have remained faithful.**

Whether you walked it or ran, it's a great feeling to cross the finish line of a race. Whether spiritual or physical, no matter how tiring our races are they are worth finishing and finishing to the best of our ability.

James 1:22-23 - And remember, it is a message to obey, not just to listen to. If you don't obey, you are only fooling yourself. For if you just listen and don't obey, it is like looking at your face in a mirror but doing nothing to improve your appearance.

You can listen to the best advice all day long, but you have to put it into practice. If you see something in your spiritual and physical mirror that needs addressed, don't ignore it.

HEBREWS 12:1-2: Therefore, since we are surrounded by such a huge crowd of witnesses to the life of faith, Let us strip off every weight that slows us down, especially the sin that so easily hinders our progress. And let us run with endurance the race that God has set before us. We do this by keeping our eyes on Jesus, on whom our faith depends from start to finish. He was willing to die a shameful death on the cross because of the joy He knew would be his afterward. Now He is seated in the place of highest honor beside God's throne in heaven.

Competitive runners wear as little as possible and what they do wear is very light. Strip off everything that slows down your spiritual race. Focus. Keep your eyes on Jesus and the finish line. Don't be looking around and getting distracted by the competition and onlookers. Don't lose your focus by focusing on others either spiritually or physically. Don't be intimidated. Run your race.

I TIMOTHY 4:6-8: If you explain this to the brothers and sisters, you will be doing your duty as a worthy servant of Christ Jesus, one who is fed by the message of faith and the true teaching you have followed. Do not waste time arguing over godless ideas and old wives tales. Spend your time and energy in training yourself for spiritual fitness. Physical exercise has some value, but spiritual exercise is much more important, for it promises a reward in both this life and the next.

If you're not moving forward you're backing up. If you're not "training" you're getting out of shape. There is no reward for being out of shape either physically or spiritually.

GALATIANS 6:1-2: Dear brothers and sisters, if another Christian is overcome by some sin, you who are godly should gently and humbly help that person back onto the right path. And be careful not to fall into the same temptation yourself. Share each other's troubles and problems, and in this way obey the law of Christ.

Help one another. Walk with each other and stand shoulder to shoulder. If a friend falls off the wagon don't run over them. Extend a hand to help them back on, but don't let them drag you off in the process.

Philippians 2:12 - Dearest friends, you were always so careful to follow my instructions when I was with you. And now that I am away you must be even more careful to put into action God's saving work in your lives, obeying God with deep reverence and fear.

The apostle Paul was obviously a personal trainer, LOL. Whether you are talking about spiritual or physical fitness, when you are taught and shown the right way you still have to live it out daily and not just when you're on the treadmill or a church pew under the supervision of your trainer or pastor.

Hebrews 13:8-9 - Jesus Christ is the same yesterday, today, and forever. So do not be attracted by strange, new ideas, Your spiritual strength comes from God's special favor, not from ceremonial rules about food, which don't help those who follow them.

Spiritually and physically there is never a shortage of the next big thing claiming to be "the way." Whether you're talking about spiritual or physical fitness, get wise counsel and do your research before jumping into something new. Truth never changes, no matter how old it is.

Some Basic Things You Need To Know

The following three journal pages are examples. The first one is the format of the journal page that is included with each day's topic. The second is an example of a more detailed nutrition journal. If you choose to make copies of the blank one that I've included and use it then you won't need to do the nutrition part of the multi section page that accompanies each day's topic. You'll notice on the nutrition sample that I have recorded the number of protein, carb, and fat grams and calories for each item eaten and totaled the calories in the far right column. This information is easily found online and in calorie count books. At the bottom is the total number of grams and calories from protein, carbs, and fat and total calories at the far right. I have also calculated the percentage of the calories for protein, carbs, and fats.

Different activity levels and lifestyles have differing caloric needs. You will need to calculate your basal metabolic rate (BMR) and your daily caloric expenditure. Your BMR is how many calories you burn in a 24 hour period if you are completely sedentary but don't sleep (watch TV without getting up for 24 hours). Your daily caloric expenditure is how many calories you actually burn after adding your lifestyle and workout habits to your BMR. So this is where you need to consult with me or a personal trainer of your choice and do your homework. Either way you do still need to do your homework. You will also need to decide on an appropriate ratio of protein, carbs, and fats. A general rule of thumb for people doing some weight training and exercising to lose weight is the 1-2-3 approach. 1 part fat, 2 parts protein, and 3 parts carbohydrate. That's 6 total parts so 6 equal parts would be approximately 311 calories using the sample page on page 16 (1866.4 / 6 = 311). That equates to 311 calories from fat, 622 (311x2) from protein, and 933 (311x3) from carbohydrates. You'll see that on the example nutrition page the actual numbers differ slightly from these, but they are certainly close enough to make the point.

In regards to the additional sample training journal page, if you find yourself needing this tool then feel free to make copies and use it. The sample workout is by no means a workout template that you should try to follow, but simply one scenario to demonstrate how to fill it out. There are countless workout routines you can apply. On the sample training journal page you will notice on each exercise that there is an intensity column. This intensity represents the level of difficulty that the particular set you just performed just gave you on a level of 1 – 10; 1 being the easiest and practically no effort and 10 being a maximum effort to get through that particular exercise. Again, consult with me or a trainer of your choice if you need some guidance in structuring something and as always, do your own homework. Read every page of the Christ Fit journal before doing anything and then let's make a game plan.

I could include a few formulas or even include a page or two of scientific information. I'm not withholding this information to entice you to patronize me or any other personal trainer. You need to understand that God designed our bodies a certain way. He invented science and he invented the science that operates our bodies. Common sense will win out so use it. You don't need the science to apply basic common sense principles that will help you become Christ Fit. If you do find yourself wanting and needing to go deeper into Christ Fit then you are going to have to be discipled and you are going to have to have someone come along side of you. The reason I don't give you a couple of pages of formulas and scientific information is because I would be giving you the bullets and the gun without proper instruction on how to combine the two. It's a process and I would love to help you and walk with you on your Christ Fit journey. We can be reached at www.ChristFitFusion.FIT or www.facebook.com/ChristFitFusion.

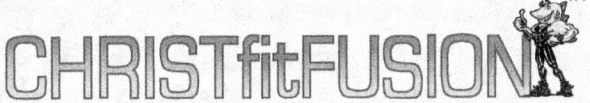

CHRISTfitFUSION™

Eat a Healthy Spiritual and Physical Diet. Exercise Spiritually and Physically. Do Them Both Consistently.

DATE: FEBRUARY 26, 2014

SPIRITUAL DIET:	PHYSICAL DIET:
6:30 A.M.– JOHN CHAPTER 3,	7:30 A.M.– 1 BOWL OF OATMEAL, 2 EGGS
NUMBERS 4, PROV. 6, PS. 75	10 A.M.– 1 CAN OF TUNA WITH CRACKERS
7:30 A.M.– RADIO– CHIP INGRAM	12 P.M.– 1 GRILLED CHICKEN BREAST, 1
8:30 A.M.– SCRIPTURE CARD ON	SMALL BOWL OF BEANS AND RICE
DESK– MARK 10: 43-45	3:30 P.M.– 1 APPLE WITH PEANUT BUTTER
5 P.M.– WORSHIP MUSIC ON	6 P.M.– 1 BAKED FISH FILLET, SALAD
DRIVE HOME (AIR 1)	(WITH RANCH LITE), BROCOLLI
6:30 P.M.– WEDNESDAY EVENING	8 P.M.– PROTIEN SHAKE
CHURCH SERVICE	

SPIRITUAL EXERCISE:	PHYSICAL EXERCISE:
READ BIBLE	30 MINUTES OF STRENGTH TRAINING
COUNSELED SON AND PRAYED	200 CRUNCHES
WITH HIM	20 MINUTE WALK WITH WIFE (MEDIUM
CHOSE WED. NIGHT CHURCH	INTENSITY)
SERVICE OVER STAYING HOME	THREW FOOTBALL WITH SON
ASKED FORGIVENESS FROM TODD	
WORSHIPED	
REPENTED– FOLLOWED RADIO	
SERMON ON DISCOURAGEMENT	
ENCOURAGED AND PRAYED WITH JIM	
RESISTED TEMPTATION TO...	

NOTES:

CHRISTfitFUSION ™

Nutrition Journal
Eat a Healthy Spiritual and Physical Diet. Exercise Spiritually and Physically. Do Them Both Consistently.

DATE: FEBRUARY 26, 2014

TIME	ITEM	QUANTITY	PROTEIN GRAMS & CALORIES	CARB GRAMS & CALORIES	FAT GRAMS & CALORIES	TOTAL CALORIES	
7:30 A.M.	OATMEAL (BROWN SUGAR)	2 PACKETS	8.6 GRAMS 34.4 CALORIES	78 GRAMS 312 CALORIES	5 GR 45 CAL	391.4	
	EGGS	2	12 G 48 C	2 G 8 C	9 G 81 C	137	
10 A.M.	TUNA W/SALSA	1 SMALL CAN (4 OZ)	22 G 88 C	0 G 0 C	0 G 0 C	88	
	CRACKERS (6 GRAIN)	1 SERVING	1.3 G 5.2 C	8.5 G 34 C	1.9 G 17.1 C	56.3	
12 P.M.	GRILLED CHICKEN BREAST	6 OZ.	35 G 140 C	0 G 0 C	2 G 18 C	158	
	PINTO BEANS	1 CUP	15.4 G 61.6 C	45 G 180 C	1 G 9 C	250.6	
	BROWN RICE	1/2 CUP	4 G 16 C	34 G 136 C	1.5 G 13.5 C	165.5	
	GREEN BEANS	1 CUP	1 G 4 C	8 G 32 C	0 G 0 C	36	
3:30 P.M.	GREEN APPLE	1	0 G 0 C	16 G 64 C	0 G 0 C	64	
	PEANUT BUTTER	1 TBSP.	4 G 16 C	3 G 12 C	8 G 72 C	100	
6 P.M.	FISH FILLET (TALAPIA)	4 OZ.	12 G 84 C	0 G 0 C	1 G 9 C	93	
	SALAD (MIXED GREENS)	1.5 CUPS	2.6 G 10.4 C	6.6 G 26.4 C	.2 G 1.8 C	38.6	
	RANCH DRESSING	2 TBSP.	0 G 0 C	1 G 4 C	7 G 63 C	67	
	BROCOLLI	1 CUP	2 G 8 C	4 G 16 C	0 G 0 C	24	
8 P.M.	PROTEIN SHAKE	2 SCOOPS	27 G 108 C	20 G 80 C	1 G 9 C	197	
		TOTALS	155.9 G 623.6 C	226.1 G 904.4 C	37.6 G 338.4 C	1866.4	
		%	623.6/1866.4 33.5%	904.4/1866.4 48.5%	338.4/1866.4 18%		

CHRISTfitFUSION™

Training Journal
Eat a Healthy Spiritual and Physical Diet. Exercise Spiritually and Physically. Do Them Both Consistently.

DATE:

	EXERCISE	REPS	WEIGHT	INTENSITY	EXERCISE	REPS	WEIGHT	INTENSITY
SET 1	LEG PRESS	15	100	3	BICEP CURL	15	15	6
SET 2	L.P.	15	150	4	B.C.	12	20	7
SET 3	L.P.	12	200	5	B.C.	12	25	8
SET 4	L.P.	10	250	7	B.C.	10	30	9
SET 5	L.P.	8	300	9	B.C.	10	35	10

	EXERCISE	REPS	WEIGHT	INTENSITY	EXERCISE	REPS	WEIGHT	INTENSITY
SET 1	LEG CURL	15	40	4	SHOULDER PRESS	15	15	3
SET 2	L.C.	15	60	6	S.P.	15	20	5
SET 3	L.C.	10	80	6	S.P.	12	25	7
SET 4	L.C.	10	90	8	S.P.	8	30	8
SET 5								

	EXERCISE	REPS	WEIGHT	INTENSITY	EXERCISE	REPS	WEIGHT	INTENSITY
SET 1	CHEST PRESS	20	60	2	AB MACHINE	50	30	5
SET 2	C.P.	15	80	3	A.M.	50	50	7
SET 3	C.P.	12	120	5	A.M.	25	70	8
SET 4	C.P.	10	150	8	A.M.	25	80	9
SET 5	C.P.	6	200	9	A.M.	20	90	10

	EXERCISE	REPS	WEIGHT	INTENSITY	EXERCISE	REPS	WEIGHT	INTENSITY
SET 1	LAT PULL	15	60	2	STRETCH	10M		
SET 2	L.P.	12	70	3				
SET 3	L.P.	10	90	5				
SET 4	L.P.	8	120	8				
SET 5	L.P.	8	150	9				

NOTES:

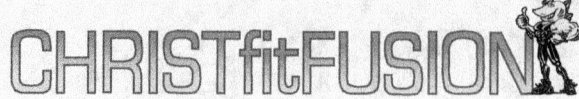

CHRISTfitFUSION™

Nutrition Journal
Eat a Healthy Spiritual and Physical Diet. Exercise Spiritually and Physically. Do Them Both Consistently.

DATE:

TIME	ITEM	QUANTITY	PROTEIN GRAMS & CALORIES	CARB GRAMS & CALORIES	FAT GRAMS & CALORIES	TOTAL CALORIES
		TOTALS				
		%				

CHRISTfitFUSION™

Training Journal

Eat a Healthy Spiritual and Physical Diet. Exercise Spiritually and Physically. Do Them Both Consistently.

DATE:

	EXERCISE	REPS	WEIGHT	INTENSITY	EXERCISE	REPS	WEIGHT	INTENSITY
SET 1								
SET 2								
SET 3								
SET 4								
SET 5								

	EXERCISE	REPS	WEIGHT	INTENSITY	EXERCISE	REPS	WEIGHT	INTENSITY
SET 1								
SET 2								
SET 3								
SET 4								
SET 5								

	EXERCISE	REPS	WEIGHT	INTENSITY	EXERCISE	REPS	WEIGHT	INTENSITY
SET 1								
SET 2								
SET 3								
SET 4								
SET 5								

	EXERCISE	REPS	WEIGHT	INTENSITY	EXERCISE	REPS	WEIGHT	INTENSITY
SET 1								
SET 2								
SET 3								
SET 4								
SET 5								

NOTES:

It's FREE! And ANY "BODY" can do it! Whether you're young, old, out of shape, disabled or have six toes. It doesn't matter. Fitness is for you and just like salvation, it's Free. It's also very simple and doesn't require a lot of fancy equipment or expensive memberships. But just like Christianity it gets way over complicated. Although the message is "simple" the follow through is one of the hardest, most challenging yet Rewarding things you'll ever do. The journey is full of trials, tribulations, pain (both good and bad), perseverance, successes, failures, plateaus, growth, and letting go of some selfish pleasures, but ultimately it leads to Victory! Are we talking about salvation or fitness here? You tell me. It applies to both.

Yes it's going to be hard, but don't think that you can't do it before you hear me out. The effort is worth it. You see, too many times the message gets soft pedaled so you will stay interested. Or there's an "easier way" with some new methodology or "miracle" solution. I'm going to be blatantly honest with you and tell you that it IS going to be tough; very tough, but you CAN do it! You NEED to do it. Listen to that voice in your head (no, not the one that sounds like Ray Romano); the one that's telling you that it's time to take that first step. Whether it's for the first time or the 100th time, draw a line in the sand and move forward. Listen to God's voice in your heart and respond to it even if responding to it means saying, "Ok, God. I don't know what to do next, please show me."

Now right up front I want you to know that I don't have a dog in this hunt. In other words, I have no personal agenda or some new workout plan, diet pill or solution to sell you. I'm not going to tell you which gym to join, which video workout to use or which "diet" to follow. To me it really doesn't matter. Does it really make a difference where you work out or which denomination you attend or which version of the Bible you read? Do something effective and do it consistently.

So how do I choose, you might ask? And yes, there are a lot of options out there. Some are good and some not so much. A good litmus test for any workout or eating plan or religion is A - Is it sustainable? B - Does it make promises that are too good to be true? And C – Does it have a proven track record? That's it!

If you need a personal trainer, fine. If you like the gym, fine. If you like sweating to the oldies, that's ok. If you need to start by walking around the block once a day, fine. Do you like "The Cabbage Diet?" Sorry, fail. What about spiritually? Do you have a church home? Is that enough? Do you read your Bible or attend a study group or are you stagnant and in need of a kick in the butt there too?

With all that in mind don't tell me that if God can inspire the writing of the Bible, speak creation into existence, and put breath in your lungs that He can't guide you into making the right decision concerning living for Him and getting Christ Fit. His ways are sustainable (sometimes difficult, but sustainable). He fulfills all His promises and never promises something He can't deliver (You may not always believe Him, but you not believing Him doesn't make it false). His track record, by the way, is impeccable.

Matthew 6:33: "But seek first the kingdom of God and his righteousness, and all these things will be added to you."

If you're living the right lifestyle the results will take care of themselves.

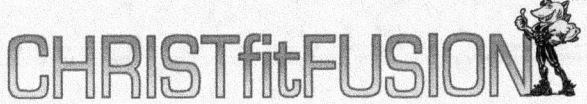

Eat a Healthy Spiritual and Physical Diet. Exercise Spiritually and Physically. Do Them Both Consistently.

DATE:

SPIRITUAL DIET: PHYSICAL DIET:

SPIRITUAL EXERCISE: PHYSICAL EXERCISE:

NOTES:

As a fitness trainer I have always encouraged clients to tell somebody when they started a fitness program with me. Whether their goal was to lose weight, get in shape for an event or just improve the way they felt in general, I challenged them to claim it and tell somebody that they knew who would occasionally ask them how they were doing with it. I wanted them to feel a sense of pressure and accountability in a positive way so that they would be less likely to flake out and quit.

Before a person gets water baptized they verbally proclaim their faith to others first. Jesus said that if anyone acknowledges Him publicly here on earth, He will openly acknowledge that person before His father in Heaven. But if anyone denies Him here on earth, He will deny that person before His father in Heaven. Hey, let's face it, if you're not ready to openly admit that Jesus is your savior then you're nowhere near ready to truly follow Him and make that "known" through baptism. So ask yourself, "Am I ready to change and be changed? Do I want to change?" If you are reading this then there's a good chance that you do or are at least thinking about it.

If the Lord is dealing with you on something or wants to change you somehow don't try to overcome it with your own strength. Lean on those who are stronger than you that God has put around you. If you struggle with food or anything else for that matter, (fill in the blank), you can try to white knuckle your way through it and yes, Jesus alone is enough and can get you through any struggle, but He also placed people in our lives for a reason and told us to bare one another's burdens and hold each other accountable. I've stopped dipping snuff before, sometimes without telling anyone (just between me and God). I've also started up again and I can tell you that the times I started again were tougher when I had told someone that I had quit. When you tell someone you instinctively don't want to let them down. When my friend, Tommy and I were training partners I knew someone was counting on me to be at the gym at a certain time. Even if I wasn't in the mood to work out I would go because I didn't want to flake out on Tommy and let him down. He was also counting on me to be there to help him and be his spotter. We helped and encouraged each other and motivated each other to get more out of our workouts than we ever could on our own.

So let the cat out of the bag. Say it. If God is prompting you in any way to address something (spiritual or physical) then tell someone, "I'm going to get into better shape. I'm going to eat healthier. I'm going to start exercising daily. I'm going to give God control of my life and I'm going to get Christ Fit." Not "I want to," "I'M GOING TO!" That makes it real and applies that positive pressure that you need. Especially when you know you can count on that person you've told to lovingly hold you accountable. Even if it's just one person, put yourself out there and engage the power of positive pressure and accountability. Who knows, you may even inspire them to go through the experience of getting Christ Fit with you.

Nothing beats personal accountability. I advise you to get some. However, journaling is a great self accountability tool as well. It has been proven that those who journal what they eat lose more weight than those who are on a "diet," but don't journal. Journal your spiritual and physical diet and exercise.

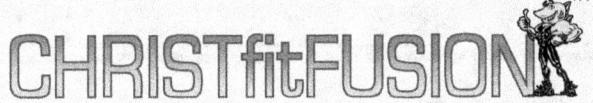

Eat a Healthy Spiritual and Physical Diet. Exercise Spiritually and Physically. Do Them Both Consistently.

DATE:

SPIRITUAL DIET: PHYSICAL DIET:

SPIRITUAL EXERCISE: PHYSICAL EXERCISE:

NOTES:

It really boils down to Choices doesn't it? You get to choose and no one is going to make your choices for you. But you do have to see the need for a change, want it, and choose to take action. So what's been holding you back; fear, apathy, misinformation? Something has. And I get it. Taking that first step towards truth can be scary.

There's a sense of uncertainty when we start something new. Will it really work? You may have seen it work for someone else, but will it work for you and what will it cost you? Results do after all, come with a price.

Have you known someone who has lost a significant amount of weight or put on 20 pounds of muscle? Have you ever seen someone seemingly transform right in front of your eyes? Maybe it wasn't physical in nature. Maybe they had a spiritual awakening of some kind; whether it was when they first came to know Jesus or something that changed in them after they already believed. But whatever it was it was as noticeable as night and day. Like "Waver Dude," as my wife and I call him. The same man walked the same route day after day and never had a pleasant expression or gesture for anyone. He was just a grumpy old guy walking down the street. I don't know what happened to him, but one day he suddenly started waving and smiling at literally every single car that passed by. If you honked and waved back you might even see him stop, beam even brighter and give you a double hand wave back. Whether he won the lottery or the love of his life died, I don't know. Something happened and whatever it was he "chose" to keep walking his same route and he chose to start doing it with a smile and enthusiasm.

It can be difficult to trust God's will for our life. What if it's not what we want or as good as we want it to be? We shouldn't doubt, but we sometimes do. It's also hard to face the truth when confronting our personal junk. Maybe you know you need to cut back on how many Cokes, beers or burgers you consume. I'm not going to say you can't have one now and then, but you know if you need to cut back just like you know if your spiritual fitness needs adjusting. But the uncertainty that surrounds making those choices to let God change you can sometimes cause you to hesitate in taking action. It's kind of like getting into the ocean or a cold pool. You put a toe in and burr! You put a foot in and wow! You step on in to above your knees and waist and then, whoa that's cold! You finally build the courage to make the choice to plunge in and for a brief moment it's exhilarating and shocking but the next thing you know you're doing it. You're swimming and enjoying it. Wouldn't it have been easier to just choose to jump in feet first in the first place? Duh. So come on. Just do it!

Make the first and most important decision and listen to God's voice and let Him guide your choices. If He's telling you to put something down or cut back then do it. Maybe it is Cokes, beers or burgers. Maybe it's your language, lust, or a gossiping tongue. If He's telling you to walk, jog or lift... read, study or volunteer then do it. Get on the track to becoming Christ Fit by listening and making the right choices.

Whether in the gym or in life there is a time to lighten the load and a time to push harder. Both are right in their own time and unproductive if applied at the wrong time. Choose wisely.

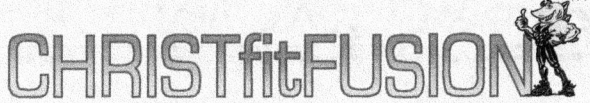

Eat a Healthy Spiritual and Physical Diet. Exercise Spiritually and Physically. Do Them Both Consistently.

DATE:

SPIRITUAL DIET: PHYSICAL DIET:

SPIRITUAL EXERCISE: PHYSICAL EXERCISE:

NOTES:

You may ask yourself "why should I get into better shape? I'm doing ok. Compared to others I'm not in 'bad' shape. There are others in worse shape than I am." That may be true, but I'm not telling you that you need to strive to be the next Arnold Schwarzenegger or Cindy Crawford. Let's get real. Not everyone is going to be a Billy Graham or a Michael Jordan. The fact is that some people truly are gifted physically and/or spiritually and although they may honestly have an extra measure of natural ability, their level of development didn't just happen. They had to be extremely disciplined in their training and go the extra mile with their diets, both physically and spiritually, in order to seemingly leap tall buildings in a single bound.

Most of us will never get a gold medal, play in the NFL or evangelize to a stadium full of people. That doesn't mean that we aren't obligated to be good stewards of the talents and bodies God has given us and do our best to take care of and develop them. Our bodies are after all the temple of the Holy Spirit, right (I Corinthians 6:19-20)? So why wouldn't we want God's temple to be as well built and spectacular as possible? Have you read the Book of Exodus? Starting in chapter 36 there is a very vivid description of the temple and altars and the extraordinary construction with all the gold and décor. It's very impressive and God gave specific instructions on just how spectacular to build it. He now inhabits us as his temple.

Now obviously we cannot literally be perfect. Not on this earth anyway. Even the most elite athletes and spiritual icons will tell you that they are far from perfect. They see themselves as always being capable of more. Always needing to work and train and hone their skills and talents. And what if they don't? Well, they start to underperform and fail to live up to their potential, don't they? If I were allowed to sit in on my own funeral one of the last things I would want to hear about myself is, "He had so much potential."

So focus on Progress rather than Perfection. That means that no matter what condition you're in (physically or spiritually) you can still improve. You'll never be perfect, but you can always make progress. Do you ever get close enough to God or get enough of Him? Heck no. There is always room for growth and improvement. We can always do better than we are doing right now. We're a work in progress from day one until we die.

So what's it going to be? Even right now you can take a quick personal inventory and something should pop out at you and it doesn't matter how small it is as long as it leads to progress. Spiritual and physical exercise; spiritual and physical diet; and doing it consistently is what it takes. Where do you need to step up right now to start making progress?

We're called to be perfect (Matt 5:48). We also know that we're a work in progress (Phil 1:6, Phil 3:12-14). Don't give up. Focus on making progress towards perfection.

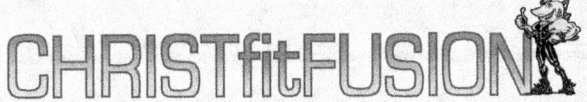

Eat a Healthy Spiritual and Physical Diet. Exercise Spiritually and Physically. Do Them Both Consistently.

DATE:

SPIRITUAL DIET: PHYSICAL DIET:

SPIRITUAL EXERCISE: PHYSICAL EXERCISE:

NOTES:

Day 5 - *Start Slow*

Don't do too much too soon. I'm not saying don't break a sweat, but listen; when you first come to Christ you're a spiritual infant. Infants need milk and basic truth. And they need it…"CONSISTENTLY" in order to grow up strong and healthy. As you get older and more mature you can handle some "mushy" foods and some deeper teachings in the Word. When you're mature then you can get after the steak and potatoes and really deep red meat of truth. If you take on too much too soon physically you only wake up paralyzed the next day unable to do anything but crawl out of bed. Similarly, you don't get saved on Sunday morning and then take on the book of Revelation all by yourself the next day... or at least you shouldn't.

I feel very certain that most of you reading this have been sore from doing something physical. I'm also fairly certain that at some point most of you have felt the kind of soreness that tells you that you way over did it.

I'm not saying don't have enthusiasm and I'm not saying don't break a sweat on your very first workout. It's even ok to be a little sore in the beginning, but this process has to be sustainable. We have the rest of our lives to work on getting Christ Fit. It doesn't all have to come together in a month or two. If a marathon runner starts off too fast in a race he burns out too quickly and doesn't finish well. If you try to take on too much weight too soon in the gym you make yourself nothing but sore and can potentially hurt yourself and experience a major setback before you ever even experience any progress.

Getting in shape is exciting. Becoming a Christian and following Christ is exciting. It's awesome to be enthusiastic and get off to a great start whether it's physical or spiritual fitness. It's fine to be pushed and stretched and challenged. Just keep in mind that getting in and staying in shape is perpetual. It's a never ending process. Think back to when you learned to ride a bike. If that's too far back to remember then think of when you taught a child to ride a bike. Things went pretty slow in the beginning. There was the learning how to get on. Learning how to sit and hold on. And even though there was probably someone holding you up and pushing you along in the beginning while you slowly learned how everything comes together you were still peddling away like you were in the Tour de France. You might not have pedaled 10 miles, but you sure felt like you were even though you were starting off slow in the grand scheme of things. You were very intentional and deliberate with everything you did. You pedaled hard to keep the bike going and there was probably someone encouraging you to pedal harder and keep pushing. Eventually you were on your own and covering more and more ground every day. Spiritually speaking your Heavenly father knows you're pushed to your max at times as you learn to ride your spiritual bicycle and He let's you be pushed and stretched, but you're still starting slow in the beginning comparatively speaking. If you told your earthly dad that you needed to slow down or that your weren't capable, he would listen if he knew you were really in a crisis. He may still push you, but he'd know if it were ok and safe to push you. So yes, start slow if you are out of shape physically or spiritually, but starting slow doesn't have to mean little effort.

Set goals and strive for them. Be reasonable. Push yourself but don't kill yourself. Get it in your head that you're in this for the long haul. And by long I mean for-e-verrr (sorry Sandlot moment).

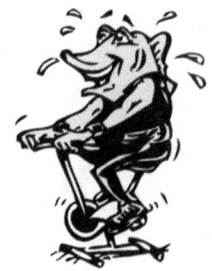

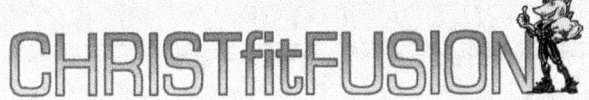

CHRISTfitFUSION™

Eat a Healthy Spiritual and Physical Diet. Exercise Spiritually and Physically. Do Them Both Consistently.

DATE:

SPIRITUAL DIET: PHYSICAL DIET:

SPIRITUAL EXERCISE: PHYSICAL EXERCISE:

NOTES:

Minor setbacks can become larger than they need to be and we can actually lose out on opportunities if we are not Christ Fit. Not being Christ Fit can cause us to miss out on certain blessings. Resist the temptation of blowing your spiritual and physical diet or missing a spiritual or physical workout.

Setbacks are absolutely going to happen. They just are. And they're going to happen in a variety of ways and at unexpected times. Some will be minor and some will be major. They're going to happen though. You will fare much better if you are Christ Fit.

In 1999 I was playing basketball with some guys from church. I jumped for a ball and got tangled up with a guy and when we landed I blew my left knee out. It hurt pretty bad for a few minutes but really just felt kind of weird. I thought I had just hyper extended it and after a few minutes I got back to my feet and started "walking it off." We started playing again and I hobbled and limped up and down the court twice trying to hang in there. Someone passed me the ball, I planted and braced with my left leg to make a cross court pass and went down like a one egg pudding. What I didn't know at the time is that I had completely severed my A.C.L., torn my M.C.L., L.C.L. and meniscus. You don't have to know what any of those are to know that it equals a major setback. For various reasons I couldn't take time off for a surgery and rehab. I rehabbed it as best I could on the fly and amazingly after a few months I was ok and functioning without a limp. I was limited (I had to leap tall buildings in a double bound) and couldn't play basketball or do other things that involved lateral movement but for the most part I was fine and could lift weights and eventually even run. At that time I was in spectacular condition and able to compensate for my injury/setback. It wasn't until about 10 years later that the beginnings of arthritis pushed me into getting surgery.

Case two. A year or so after injuring my knee I bumped into the family of a guy I had gone to high school with. The story is too long to tell here, but it was totally a divine appointment. It turned out that the guy was in need of a kidney. After several months and several tests I ended up donating a kidney to this guy and God saved his life. Even though that was a voluntary setback it was still a setback and required a recovery. But again, being fit and in good shape helped make the road to recovery much shorter and honestly it required being in relatively good health in the first place just to be able to do the surgery. Although it was a setback it's one that I was glad to participate in and am glad I was in a position to do it.

Living a Christ Fit lifestyle will definitely help you weather the storms of life. Whether a simple cold, a major injury, a spiritual attack or catastrophe, you really can't afford not to be Christ Fit. Just think about all you stand to lose out on if you're not at least somewhat fit. Even simple things like playing ball with kids and carrying groceries make it worth it (I personally take pride in being able to carry my weight in groceries and turn a 3 tripper from the car to the house into 1). For some of my older clients being fit has meant independence and lowering the risk of a fall and being more durable in case they did fall. But there are even bigger dangers as well. Setbacks are going to happen. You're going to struggle with sin. Family members are going to die. You need to start getting Christ Fit if you aren't already.

Not everyone is going to have the opportunity to donate an organ, but everyone is going to have the opportunity to be used by God one way or another. I don't know what that is for you and you may not know either. The scary thing is that you may never know unless you're Christ Fit. The fact of the matter is that you're here for a reason and God uses people every day to accomplish his purposes. He uses people to share their faith, teach Sunday school, go on missions trips, give to the needy, love on children and plant churches. The list is endless and includes small roles and Billy Graham roles. But even Billy Graham had helpers that weren't in the spot light.

No matter what setbacks are headed your way. No matter what assignments God has planned for you. You can't afford not to be Christ Fit.

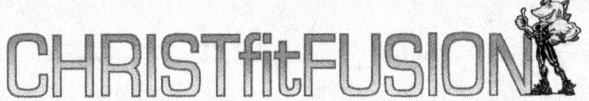

Eat a Healthy Spiritual and Physical Diet. Exercise Spiritually and Physically. Do Them Both Consistently.

DATE:

SPIRITUAL DIET: PHYSICAL DIET:

SPIRITUAL EXERCISE: PHYSICAL EXERCISE:

NOTES:

Just as important as a good workout program is the time needed to recover from it. The callus effect is your body adapting to stress and turning blisters/trauma to calluses (explained in more detail on Day 27- No Pain No Gain). A workout causes trauma to your body so it needs time to recover from that trauma and adapt to that stress. Traumatizing/breaking down already broken down muscle tissue is counterproductive. How much recovery time differs from person to person but it is a must for everyone.

Over and over again if you pay attention you'll see some people doing the same thing day in and day out (I'm a professional people watcher). There's the guy that if he steps foot in the gym, whether once a week or 7 days a week, he's going to do bicep curls. There's the gal that no matter what, is going to do the butt master and the crunch machine (that's an ab exercise, not where you get your chocolate crunch bar). Even if their biceps and booty cheeks look pretty good you'll notice over time they never get any bigger, better, firmer, or stronger. They're stagnant and plateaued.

Your body has to have recovery time to improve and be its best. You can still do daily exercise, but you need to be strategic. If you're doing resistance training, don't do the same body parts every day. You could do legs one day, chest and triceps the next day, back and biceps the next day and by then your legs have had time to recover and you can do them again. That's just one example. There are 100's of ways to structure your routine. If you're walking/jogging you don't need to set a personal best record every time. Generally speaking if your muscles are sore then you're still recovering. That applies to both resistance training and cardio. So can you walk/jog every day? Sure. But if you're still a little sore you may need to have an easy day where you're just working out the soreness and not breaking down more muscle tissue. Can you do resistance training every day? Sure. But if a body part is still a little sore you don't need to do as much as your previous workout with that particular body part (if any at all). Do enough to work out some soreness but don't traumatize your muscles any more than they already are. Recover.

But what about the person who runs 6 miles a day and doesn't get sore? They even run pretty hard every day. Well, they are what you call "in shape." Their body has adapted to a continuous stress (callouses effect). Their body has developed the ability to recover faster and operate more efficiently. But even they will ease up as they approach the day of a 10k road race. And even they, as hard as they train, when they push extra hard (more than the normal stress that they usually endure) can still get "blisters" (soreness) and need recovery time. Now recovery time doesn't mean take a month off either. At the end of a season in any given sport an athlete will usually have a little down time to recover from the grueling season. But even when they take some down time or a week or two off it's not long before they're moving their bodies a little bit and doing something light and easy.

So do we ever need to recover spiritually? I think so. I know pastors and others in ministry do. They give and study their brains out and pour into people and need to recover from all that spiritual exercise. I even needed a break every once in a while during the writing of this journal. So if you find yourself getting Christ Fit and starting to serve and volunteer or whatever; don't forget to recover when you need it. Don't take a spiritual vacation, but every now and then take some recovery and just read your Bible for yourself. Recovery time is an essential part of being balanced and Christ Fit otherwise you can end up with spiritual blisters that manifest themselves as bitterness, irritability, resentment and spiritual burn out.

Genesis 2:2: "On the seventh day God had finished His work of creation, so He rested from all His work."

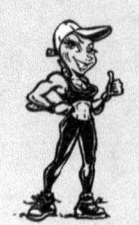

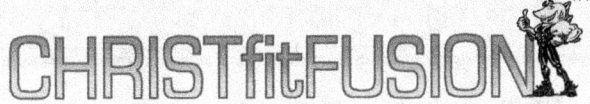

Eat a Healthy Spiritual and Physical Diet. Exercise Spiritually and Physically. Do Them Both Consistently.

DATE:

SPIRITUAL DIET: PHYSICAL DIET:

SPIRITUAL EXERCISE: PHYSICAL EXERCISE:

NOTES:

Don't "diet." Just eat right. Diets don't work! It's a multimillion dollar marketing industry. That's why there's a new one every other week. If we are living a fitness lifestyle the results will happen. It's not going to happen overnight, but it will happen. Our transformation, whether physical or spiritual is a process. The way it happens is a process. That process involves following some fundamental principles rather than chasing every new philosophy that comes around. Jesus has never changed and neither has common sense eating habits.

Diets, according to various studies, have a failure rate of 95% - 99%. A failed diet is nothing more than losing weight, but failing to keep it off permanently.

Why do "diets" fail? Diets fail because most are unsustainable. Also, there is usually an unhealthy perspective and mind set of "losing weight" and not changing a lifestyle permanently. The goal of a "diet" should be to lose fat, not just weight, and to keep it off and consistently improve. The problem with most diets is that the weight loss includes muscle weight which in turns slows down your metabolic rate (the rate at which you burn calories) and makes you susceptible to putting weight back on, which if you're not working out and eating healthy is all fat and you end up back at your old weight or more and with a higher percentage of body fat and the cycle starts all over again. Hmm. Sounds kind of like when Jesus said that a demon will return with 7 more (Matthew 12: 43-45). To permanently lose body fat requires a lifestyle not a diet. When you do lose fat you can't raise your hands in victory and go back to your old ways that got you fat in the first place. A lifestyle is just that; a style of life that you live day in a day out forever. So when you have that perspective you have your whole life to get in shape. So what's the hurry? It's a process. To be successful in your diet you have to be inspired, not just motivated. You have to change the way you think, re-educate your habits, and commit to a lifestyle. Motivation is all about psyching yourself up to do something that you think you should or that you're supposed to do. Being inspired is more about a calling and doing something "in spirit." It's being divinely influenced.

Just like with dieting we can yo-yo spiritually. We can cut out spiritual sugars, eat more spiritual protein, and drop a few sin pounds. Unless we are living a healthy lifestyle though, we put it right back on. It can be very depressing and give us a "what's the use" mentality. The Matthew 12: 43-45 effect again.

It's all about a sustainable, healthy, balanced lifestyle. We have got to let God's spirit inspire us and change our thought process. If you've developed some bad spiritual and physical dietary habits because of life's experiences then so be it, but let God change you and break the cycle. If we are living the right lifestyle and letting God change us over time the results will happen, but we have to live it daily for the rest of our lives to be Christ Fit.

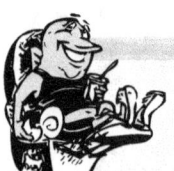

I Thessalonians 5:17-18: "Never stop praying. Be thankful in all circumstances, for this is God's will for you who belong to Christ Jesus."

We aren't called to "gorge" on God's word or pray 24 hours a day, but we are essentially told to "graze" on it. Our bodies of course work so much better when we graze on food rather than gorge once or twice a day. Not on pizza or sugar of course, but when we have a steady consumption in small doses of healthy nutrition (spiritually and physically) our spirit and bodies naturally speed up their metabolism, crave more of the good stuff and get healthier and fitter.

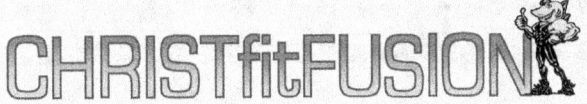

CHRISTfitFUSION™

Eat a Healthy Spiritual and Physical Diet. Exercise Spiritually and Physically. Do Them Both Consistently.

DATE:

SPIRITUAL DIET: PHYSICAL DIET:

SPIRITUAL EXERCISE: PHYSICAL EXERCISE:

NOTES:

In case you haven't caught on yet... Christ Fit is built on a platform of eating a "healthy" spiritual and physical diet, getting "healthy" spiritual and physical exercise, and doing them both consistently. That's it, simple! Is it easy? Of course it's not. If it were, everyone would be Christ Fit. But... the gate is narrow... I guess if the gate is "narrow" that's one good reason to get Christ Fit, right? So when it comes to diet and exercise there are three basic components: Frequency, Healthy, and Portion Control.

DIET:

Frequency: I'm not going to even start to explain the body's metabolism and all the science. Look it up. The Bible says work out your own salvation... So go read a fitness book, or medical or science journal if you don't believe me, but the grazing approach is very well known and truly the only way to go. You have to eat breakfast, a snack, lunch, a snack, and dinner; and then a snack involving ice cream right before bed. Yummo! The body requires constant healthy fuel to function at peak performance. You don't ask your vehicle to run on empty with the promise that you'll fill it up later do you? It doesn't work. You're body doesn't function properly when it is deprived of nutrition.

Healthy: You have to put the right kind of fuel in your body. Grazing (Eating smaller amounts more frequently) on junk food will not work any better than not eating enough. If you have pop tarts for breakfast, a candy bar for a snack, pizza for lunch, etc. then you're going to be unfit regardless of the grazing principle. You can't consistently put junk in your body spiritually or physically and be Christ Fit.

Consistency: Having a good day once a week for an entire year is consistent but consistently wrong. Stringing together a few good days in a row every month is consistent, but won't get you anywhere. I get the occasional mess up or blown day, but your general day in and day out routine has got to be consistently healthy in order to make any progress.

So with frequency, healthy, and consistency in mind, take a look at your "Spiritual Diet." How many days a week do you eat a spiritual breakfast? For many it's just one (Sunday Morning). For many, maybe even you, Sunday morning is the "ONLY" spiritual meal of the entire week. If that is you then you are starving to death spiritually. In order to be Christ Fit you need that spiritual breakfast every morning and you need to graze throughout the day. It's not nearly as hard as you might think either. Get in the Word before you leave the house (even if it's just a Proverb for the day), catch a teaching on the radio or podcast on the way to work, read a five minute daily devotional during lunch, etc. It's not that hard. It just takes commitment.

And just as important is "What" we feed on spiritually; If you put junk in your mind the way you put junk in your stomach you're going to get more and more spiritually unhealthy. You have to graze on the right stuff and you have to do it consistently. If you wonder why you feel spiritually weak sometimes then consider your diet. Your healthy spiritual diet has to be consistent if you want to be Christ Fit.

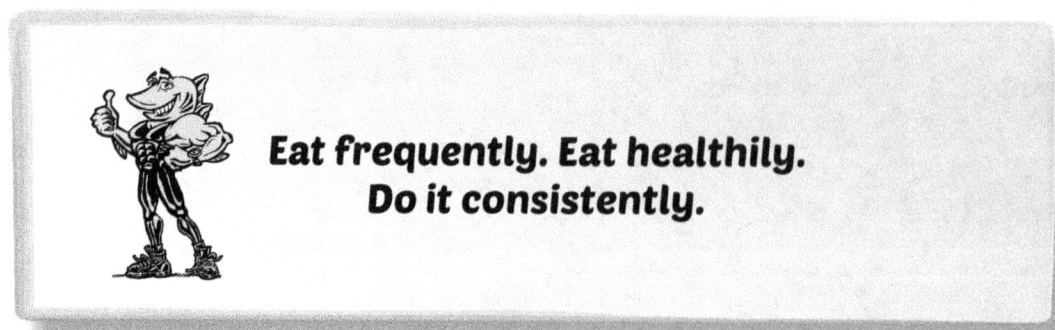

**Eat frequently. Eat healthily.
Do it consistently.**

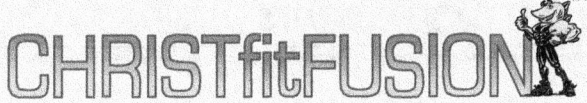

CHRISTfitFUSION™

Eat a Healthy Spiritual and Physical Diet. Exercise Spiritually and Physically. Do Them Both Consistently.

DATE:

SPIRITUAL DIET: PHYSICAL DIET:

SPIRITUAL EXERCISE: PHYSICAL EXERCISE:

NOTES:

37

EXERCISE

Frequency: You can't workout once a week and expect to get in shape. You can't workout one week out of the month and expect to get in shape. You can't kill it for three months out of the year and succeed. You absolutely must exercise frequently. I suggest doing something every day. Even if you have an easy day once or twice a week and just go fishing or play backyard ball with your kids or stroll through the park with your sweetheart, do something. If on a workout day you end up only having 15 minutes then make the most of it, but don't "not workout." Just like the scriptures that tell us to pray without ceasing and to be continuously filled with the spirit… that's frequency. Make spiritual and physical fitness part of your daily lifestyle. I even played 4-square with my family once and called it my exercise for the day.

Healthy: Yes, there is such a thing as unhealthy exercise. Taking on too much too soon, pushing too hard for your ability, spending too many hours in the gym at one time (over training) can be unhealthy. Just like with diet and the grazing principle; short, small (20 – 30 minute) intense workouts are ideal. You could make a case that they are the best.

You can have unhealthy spiritual exercise as well. Wanting to serve in church is great. Wanting to help people out all the time is nice. But if you're not called to do it; if you take on more than you're supposed to; you'll find yourself burned out and unproductive.

Exercise spiritually and physically, but do it healthily.

Consistency: Just like with diet; once a day each week is consistent. January through February every year is consistent, but whether physically or spiritually, neither is productive.

Find something that is challenging and also sustainable. Over time you will have to push harder to challenge yourself, but the key is to do something every day of every week of every year over and over again. Consistency.

Healthy habits can be hard to develop. Taking that first step is often daunting. It's almost as if you're looking up a mountain that you have to climb and thinking that you just can't make it to the top. But you can. Just take it one step at a time. I know it's hard. Trust me, I really do. Is it easy to get up earlier in the morning? Fitting time in during a lunch hour? Making time during the evening after a long day? Heck No. Not at first anyway. But here's the deal. You already have BAD habits! For the first few days (or months for some of you) you may have to throw yourself out of bed. Eventually though, your body will not feel right if you do not get your workout or God time in… You'll do it whether you feel like it or not. You'll feel strange and like something is out of place if you don't. You'll miss those endorphins and spiritual highs.

So develop some healthy habits. Even if it's just a chapter a day or a few crunches at bed time to start out with. Take some first steps up that mountain and get on your way to becoming Christ Fit.

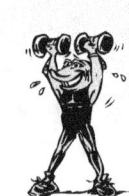

**Exercise frequently. Exercise healthily.
Do it consistently.**

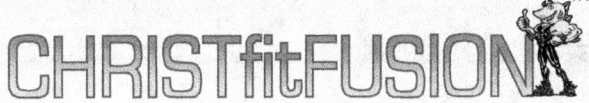

Eat a Healthy Spiritual and Physical Diet. Exercise Spiritually and Physically. Do Them Both Consistently.

DATE:

SPIRITUAL DIET: PHYSICAL DIET:

SPIRITUAL EXERCISE: PHYSICAL EXERCISE:

NOTES:

There is no substitute for the real thing. The only reason we crave substitutes is because we are missing enough of the real deal. Even when we're deceived into buying into a counterfeit, thinking it's the real thing, ultimately the reason we're using the substitute is because we don't have enough of the real thing in us to know we're being tricked.

It's like this; most of us would agree that Diet Coke isn't "good" for us. It has less sugar and calories than regular Coke, but it still has no nutritional value. We get thirsty, we want to quench it, we reach for the Diet Coke because it's "healthier" than Coke. Hey dummy, if you're thirsty your body's craving water. If you had enough water in you, you wouldn't crave Coke or the Diet Coke in the first place. On a side note, I have to admit that I love Coke and once in a while I crave one no matter how much water I've had. And if I'm going to have one it's going to be a real one; not any of that "diet" mess. And yes it's ok to have a Coke now and then. It just can't be part of our daily lifestyle. Fill in the blank with any food substitute that you struggle with. If you're not grazing and filling your body with real nutrition you're going to crave the substitutes and you're most likely going to overdo it.

Of course there's the spiritual side of things. What about our spiritual nutrition? First of all, are you even getting any or are you living off of spiritual chocolate frosted sugar bombs and deep fried Twinkies? If you're not getting any or enough spiritual nutrition you may not even know that you're falling for a substitute.

What are you substituting for spiritual fitness: work, partying, shopping, a hobby, addiction, or even too many weekend soccer games? Fill in your own blanks. You're craving something and you don't even know it. You're craving real spiritual nutrition. The substitutes can certainly be tasty. I'll admit that. They can be very tempting even on the best of days, just like the Coke. But keep a steady flow of spiritual nutrition coming in. Fill up on it so you won't have room for the junk. You'll find the cravings are a lot more manageable and you'll find that you become more disciplined, stronger and Christ Fit.

Spiritually and Physically, there is no substitute that is better for you than the real thing.

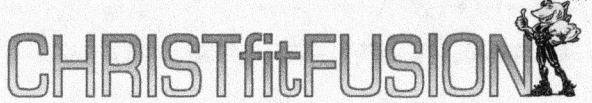

Eat a Healthy Spiritual and Physical Diet. Exercise Spiritually and Physically. Do Them Both Consistently.

DATE:

SPIRITUAL DIET: PHYSICAL DIET:

SPIRITUAL EXERCISE: PHYSICAL EXERCISE:

NOTES:

Day 12 - *Metabolism: Fire It Up*

One of the keys to losing body fat is a fast metabolism. There are various factors that impact our metabolism. Some positive factors that help speed it up include: gaining muscle, being hydrated, exercise, healthy macro nutrients (Protein, Carbs, and Fats), and micro nutrients (Vitamins & Minerals). There are also negative influences on metabolism: sugars and other empty calories, starving (not eating enough causes your body to go into self-preservation mode and slow its metabolism down as a survival mechanism), high body fat, dehydration, and being sedentary.

It's really very simple. Think of a camp fire. When you start putting the right factors in place your metabolism becomes like a roaring camp fire. The more healthy fuel you put on it the hotter it gets. The more junk you throw on it the smaller it gets or it burns toxic. One of the worst things you can do to a fire is to deprive it of fuel. It'll go out. When you start exercising and building your muscles, drinking water, and putting healthy nutrition in your body, your fire burns hot. You'll also be able to tell when a wet log or dirty diaper has been thrown on. You won't feel so great. Your fire will dwindle, stink, and not be hot. The good news is that a hot enough fire can consume a wet log or a dirty diaper once in a while. It just can't live on it.

Our spiritual metabolism is even more important and works in much the same way. If our spiritual fire is smoldering or burning low we need to adjust what we're putting on it or failing to put on it. Stoke that fire and get it burning hot. No matter how your fire is burning at the moment you can get it burning hot or even hotter if it's already healthy.

Think about this. Whether you're building a fire from scratch or have a fire that has been burning but is getting low because of a lack of attention you start with kindling. You can't start a fire or stoke one up by using big logs alone. You'll just snuff the whole thing out. You have to put little bits of paper, straw, and twigs on it. Once that catches you can add a few sticks that are a little bigger. As the fire builds up you can put on bigger and bigger logs.

So if your spiritual and/or physical fire is down to a bed of coals it may not be wise to try to devour an entire full body hard core workout physically or engulf an entire book of the Bible spiritually. Just start with some little bits of kindling and build up. You can handle a little bit of exercise and a few key scriptures. The key is to put little bits of healthy fuel on your fire and progressively build up to a roaring fire. When your fire gets hot and is burning big you can devour the big logs.

So fire it up. Put the right fuel on the fire, stop throwing crap on there and do this. The hotter it gets, the hotter you'll want it and the more you'll crave the healthy fuel.

Keys To A Hot Spiritual and Physical Fire/Metabolism:

Feed it frequently.
Don't let it get low or go out.
Put smaller logs on it.
Put healthy fuel on it.
Avoid putting trash or toxic logs on it.

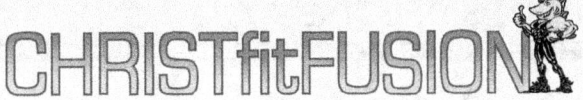

Eat a Healthy Spiritual and Physical Diet. Exercise Spiritually and Physically. Do Them Both Consistently.

DATE:

SPIRITUAL DIET: PHYSICAL DIET:

SPIRITUAL EXERCISE: PHYSICAL EXERCISE:

NOTES:

Christ Fit is all about balance and sustainability; eating a healthy spiritual and physical diet, exercising and training spiritually and physically and doing them both consistently. To do anything consistently it has to be sustainable, otherwise you just burn out. Of all the options out there what is sustainable? Most "diets" and "exercise programs" are unsustainable so you usually end up quitting and starting several times or moving on in search of the next holy grail of fitness. I'm all about eating plenty of protein, but a protein only or "no carb" diet just isn't the answer. It's unsustainable. Our bodies need carbs. It's our most readily available source of energy and necessary for brain function as well. We're designed to run on them. On the flip side of that coin is that excess carbs (any excess calories for that matter) are stored as fat. There's got to be balance.

There are plenty of exercise programs and routines out there. Some are sustainable and some are junk. Some are sustainable once you're in shape, but are not sustainable for getting into shape. It's easy to get lured by the chiseled abs and lean bodies on the infomercial hard bodies. If the truth be told the devil masquerades as an angel of light and most of those hard bodies are doing a heck of a lot more than the "magic bullet" they are promoting.

I'm willing to bet that you can't name one person that has gotten in shape and stayed in shape for more than 5 years that will give credit to a TV infomercial promoting a diet or exercise routine. Think about it. Have you ever heard of a long time in shape person say, "I owe it all to the 'Gazelle,' the 'Ab Roller,' or 'Atkins?'" You don't hear that. Long time in shape people find their way by working out their own salvation and find a healthy balance with eating and exercise.

What about spiritual fitness? No doubt diet and exercise require hard work and discipline even when there is balance. So does spiritual fitness. It's going to be hard; that's just a fact, but at least when there's balance there can be sustainability.

So are you on the "church only" / "Starvation Diet?" Have you tried the spiritual P90X to the 100th power exercise program and sweated your spiritual sports bra or jock off? What about the ever popular "I do all of it – a very well balanced overdose of everything" program?

Balance and sustainability are crucial. We need protein, carbs, and even fat. We need to hear the Word at church and have quite time in the Word and prayer time alone. We need fellowship. We need to serve and sometimes be humble to let others serve us. We need every aspect of spiritual fitness to be Christ Fit, but too much of one thing and not enough of the other is unbalanced and unsustainable.

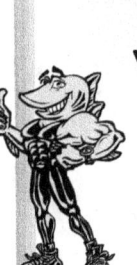

You need a healthy balance of spiritual and physical diet and exercise to be Christ Fit.

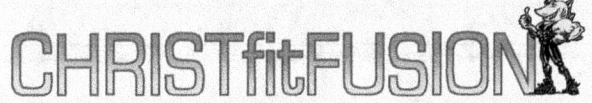

Eat a Healthy Spiritual and Physical Diet. Exercise Spiritually and Physically. Do Them Both Consistently.

DATE:

SPIRITUAL DIET: PHYSICAL DIET:

SPIRITUAL EXERCISE: PHYSICAL EXERCISE:

NOTES:

Day 14 - Supplements

Supplement: A Noun: 1). Something added to complete a thing, supply a deficiency, or reinforce or extend a whole. 2). A part added to a book, document etc., to supply additional or later information, correct errors or the like. 3). A part, usually of special character, issued as an additional feature of a newspaper or other periodical (www.thefreedictionary.com).

Supplements are great. I, personally, am a big fan. It is virtually impossible to get enough vitamins and minerals in our diet without them. If you're not already taking a high quality multi-vitamin supplement I highly recommend it. Remember, we need vitamins for basic bodily functions, metabolism, and overall health. They're extremely important and practically a necessity to supplement if you want to get enough vitamins and minerals in your diet.

Now aside from vitamins, there's protein powder and amino acids to make you stronger and supplements to speed up your metabolism and make you skinny. There's supplements for joint health, supplements for memory, supplements to help you sleep, some to help your sex life, and some will even make your farts smell pretty (I wish).

If you need a supplement use it. But keep in mind it's a supplement; not a replacement for the real thing. I love a good protein shake as much as anybody. It's quick, easy, transportable, tastey, and helps me get my needed amount of protein in without having to eat my weight in tuna. If shakes were all I consumed, I'd certainly get plenty of protein and I could probably live off of them as long as I was willing to wear a diaper full time. It's not worth it. It's a great supplement, but you can't use it to replace the real thing. Real food has too much value.

Way too many people trying to lose weight use supplements and expect the supplement to do the work for them. And to be honest they're more concerned with "losing weight" and "looking" in better shape than living a lifestyle that gets them healthy.

I also recommend and personally enjoy spiritual supplements. There are many good ones and many that have truly helped me with my spiritual fitness. My wife and I both love good books, conferences, retreats, etc., but there is no replacing God's one true living Word, the Bible. As simple and "boring" as it may seem you just can't get around the necessity for true fundamentals. Like trying to live off protein shakes it is impossible to live off spiritual supplements alone. For me it goes down like this sometimes. Life gets busy. I have some late nights. I sleep in till 5:30 and miss my alone time with God. I keep up with my supplements though and catch a good sermon on the radio. Maybe even 3 or 4 of them. Life goes on like this for a few days and I'm getting loads of awesome teaching from fantastic pastors and teachers. I'm getting my verse of the day texts ect., but I'm not getting my daily one on one quiet time with God and time in His word. Even though I'm getting some healthy spiritual supplementation there are some key nutrients missing. It's during those times that I start to get a little spiritually weak and vulnerable to sin, which drives me back to the fundamentals. Eat a healthy spiritual and physical diet. Exercise spiritually and physically. Do them both consistently.

It's fine to supplement, but the thing that you add to a thing can't be the main thing.

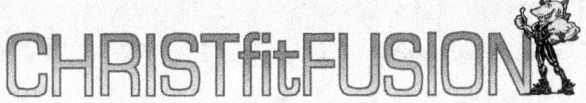

CHRISTfitFUSION™

Eat a Healthy Spiritual and Physical Diet. Exercise Spiritually and Physically. Do Them Both Consistently.

DATE:

SPIRITUAL DIET: PHYSICAL DIET:

SPIRITUAL EXERCISE: PHYSICAL EXERCISE:

NOTES:

Day 15 - *Thrive or Survive*

There's a tremendous contrast between thriving and surviving. So what makes the difference between the two? Whether talking about humans, plants, animals or even in the "teenage" kingdom, some seem to thrive and some just barely survive. Granted, there are times that we all go into survival mode to some degree and sometimes those periods of surviving seem to last an eternity, but even in those times of survival we can still ultimately thrive.

In a race there are those that sometimes jump out in front and although they lead and appear to thrive there comes a time when they appear to be just trying to survive the pace that they've set. The movie Running Brave is the story of Billy Mills, a Lakota Sioux Indian that won the 1964 Olympic 10,000 meter race in Japan. His entire story is remarkable and one of surviving and eventually thriving. He was a virtual no name going into the event. He qualified with a time almost a minute slower than his competitors and even had to borrow shoes for the race. Ron Clarke from Australia and Mohamed Gammoudi form Tunisia were expected to place first and second. Third was up to the other 34 runners in the field. It was a very dramatic race and from the start Clarke set the tone. Mills did manage to survive and hang with the leaders and with one lap to go it was Clarke, Gammoudi, and Mills. Mills took a slight and very brief lead. Clarke bumped Mills as they passed a slower runner and then Gammoudi wedged his way between both of them for the lead. Mills had been knocked off balance and lost a lot of ground.

Coming out of the last turn Clarke was chasing Gammoudi in a seemingly two man race for the win. Mills was boxed in with lap traffic and out of contention. He pulled out to lane four and out of nowhere hit the jets like a sprinter, passed Clarke and Gammoudi and won pulling away with a time of 28:24.4, almost 50 seconds faster than he had ever run before. One of the Japanese officials came up to him after the race and asked him over and over again, "Who are you? Who are you?" He had just set a new Olympic record.

I can tell you that there is no greater high than to run your race in Christ and cross that finish line thriving. One of my Billy Mills moments occurred at boot camp when I was 17. I was at Ft. Benning Georgia and we were doing our P.T. test. One of the events was the two mile run. All of the companies in our battalion were running together in three heats. I was in the fast heat and although it was only for personal time and not a "race" it may as well have been the Olympics for me. Anytime you get guys doing the same thing at the same time it's a competition and there has to be a winner. The drill sergeants wanted bragging rights, and all of the privates wanted their company's runner to be the best. I knew who the expected winners were and I knew that I was not one of them. As we crossed the start/finish line with one lap to go I was struggling to keep up with the leaders. I was a few seconds behind, but surviving. As we ran past the other privates watching us run I caught a few words that I don't think were even intended for me to hear. Fisher, one of my buddies, said to another guy, "Nokes is going to catch them." That was all it took and something inside me swelled. The track was ½ mile around with woods in the infield. As we disappeared around turn one it was me chasing a few other guys. No cheering and no witnesses; just a lonely track and the choice to make excuses or survive. As we hit the final turn all the drill sergeants were there to encourage us with yelling, cursing insults and threats to our lives if we didn't win. As we rounded the final turn there were our fellow privates down at the finish line doing everything they could to inspire us. That was the longest 200 meters in the world. I was in second place by this time and the guy I was trying to catch seemed like an 8 foot avatar out of a sci-fi movie. But I did it. I don't know how, but I did it. I won.

We are in a spiritual race. What will make the difference in us thriving or surviving? Eating a healthy spiritual and physical diet; exercising and training spiritually and physically; and doing them both consistently. Even then there is only so much that training can do. You've sometimes got to have something extra. That ability to dig deep and find that spirit inside of you that pushes you to do the seemingly impossible. It's the eye of the tiger mentality. I'm not saying that we can do this in and of ourselves. It's totally a God thing, but it's there and it's accessible. You just have to tap into it. I want to encourage you. Wherever you're at in your race, as long as you still have breath in your lungs it's not over and you can still finish well. You can do it.

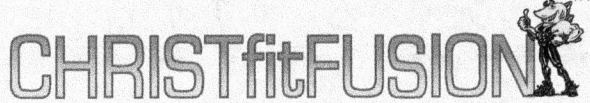

CHRISTfitFUSION™

Eat a Healthy Spiritual and Physical Diet. Exercise Spiritually and Physically. Do Them Both Consistently.

DATE:

SPIRITUAL DIET: PHYSICAL DIET:

SPIRITUAL EXERCISE: PHYSICAL EXERCISE:

NOTES:

Day 16 - *Targeting*

Spiritually and physically we all have problem areas. I'm going to give you the secret to targeting any body part and any specific sin or stronghold in your life. Whether you have triceps that wave good bye long after the rest of you stops or you're tangled up in a perpetual merry go round of sin and repentance with the same issue there is a sure fired guaranteed way to target those pesky problem areas.

The problem for most folks is that they aim at the wrong target and hit it every time. The "secret" is this; "Stop Targeting!" Sorry if you're let down, but it's going to take a lot more than extra reps on the butt blaster to tone your buns and it's going to take a lot more than will power and trying harder to get that speck out of your eye. My workout partner back in the day had great abs. The trouble was that you couldn't see them. You could feel them through the body fat covering them and he could do ab exercises all day long but that six pack just never popped. The total package with nutrition and lifestyle just wasn't there to allow the fat to shrink enough to reveal his washboard stomach. The same will be true for any body part or sin in our lives.

So what do we do when we have a bona fide problem area that needs attention? We see it. We're conscious of it and we know we need to deal with it, but what do we do? I certainly don't want to lead you to believe that we don't need to address our junk. When we have a gut (or a sin...) our instinct is to do crunches or get on some machine that targets that area. The machine of choice may not be counterproductive, but it is usually a "waist" of time if that's where you put most of your focus. There are a lot of silly looking exercises and machines that have the appearance of being beneficial, but do little to help. Similarly you can target a sin and still be just as fat spiritually as if you didn't even try to handle it.

Eat a healthy spiritual and physical diet. Exercise spiritually and physically. Do them both consistently. That's the secret. If you are living the right lifestyle the results will take care of themselves.

We must have a spiritual perspective on everything. The devil and his punk angels will attack wherever they can to get you out of God's will. Even with food and unhealthy lifestyle. Anything to get you to focus on you (even if negatively). So whatever we are dealing with let's get back to basics and target our lifestyle. Matthew 6:33 - Seek first the kingdom of God and everything will be added to you. Everything means everything.

So spend some quiet time with God. Talk to Him and more importantly take time to listen to Him. Get in His Word. Get honest with Him. Eat healthy foods in the right amount. Exercise your entire body. Do your exercises that you like (spiritually and physically) but don't neglect the hard ones that are more challenging and not as much fun. Squats hurt, but they are good for the entire body. Fasting is uncomfortable but it allows God to speak into your life. If you are spending quality time with God and getting a "balanced" diet spiritually and physically He is going to give you the nudge, push, and strength to deal with your junk. If your focus is on your junk and you are just trying harder to overcome it your focus will not be on Jesus. If your focus is on Jesus and if you obey (key word) His promptings you're going to deal with the junk naturally. He's going to deal with it with you. Ask Him to make His will your will and then listen for what He puts in your heart. (I John 5:14-15 - And we are confident that He hears us whenever we ask for anything that pleases Him. And since we know He hears us when we make our requests, we also know that He will give us what we ask for).

Anytime I start to notice something in the mirror that I don't like I can look at my training journal and see where I have been weak with my training or diet and why I am having a problem. Whenever I look into my spiritual mirror and see something I don't like or when I start to slip where I haven't been tempted in a long time I can look at my spiritual training journal and see where I've gotten off. It's usually because I've been doing some easy spiritual exercises like catching a sermon on the radio while I drive (good stuff) while neglecting some of the more challenging ones like cutting out specific time to get with God in a quite place to let Him address me personally and fill me up with His spirit.

Unhealthiness, being overweight, sin of any kind are manifestations of a problem. They are not in and of themselves the issue. So address the root of the plant. Not just its fruit.

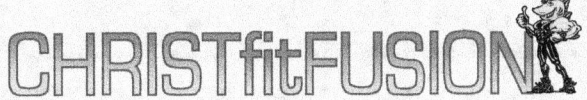

CHRISTfitFUSION™

Eat a Healthy Spiritual and Physical Diet. Exercise Spiritually and Physically. Do Them Both Consistently.

DATE:

SPIRITUAL DIET: PHYSICAL DIET:

SPIRITUAL EXERCISE: PHYSICAL EXERCISE:

NOTES:

Day 17 - Only One Way?

Although there is only one way to Heaven, there are still options and choices to make. Have you ever known a person who was extraordinarily fit in one way or another? Maybe they were an excellent endurance runner, basketball player or someone who was extremely strong. Three distinctly fit people, but in different ways. All three have to train and discipline their bodies in order to be fit in their unique way, but they are all fit. The strong person may not be able to keep up with the endurance runner in a marathon, but he can be just as fit with equally healthy blood pressure, heart rate, cholesterol, body fat percentage etc. Both athletes have to fuel their bodies with the right nutrition and exercise appropriately, but they also have an area of expertise which requires specific diet and training. The same holds true with our "spiritual fitness." We all need the same basic elements, "living water," "spiritual food" from the Word, fellowship, prayer etc. but at the same time, once we achieve a general level of spiritual fitness we too can specialize in a particular discipline. Some Christians are especially fit in their eschatology. Some are gifted in their ability to teach and still others are gifted with a special ability to counsel or minister in other ways. All can be just as spiritually fit, but with a specific expertise just like athletes.

Regardless of a person's area of mastery we all have to start somewhere; the beginning. Every professional or elite athlete out there started off dropping the ball, getting winded and generally missing the mark somehow. They had to master the basics and be disciplined early on in their initial training to develop the skills to be able to eventually train harder and more specifically for their professional pursuits. They also learned where they were most gifted and had the most propensities for success. I'm sure it didn't take Shaquille O'neal long to determine that he wasn't going to be an elite gymnast. Generally speaking you can just tell by looking, that a person is or isn't cut out for a particular genre of sports.

It is impossible to tell just by looking at a person's physical appearance what their spiritual gifts are, but they are there nonetheless. No matter what our spiritual gifts are, like the Billy Grahams of the world, we must start somewhere - The beginning. We must go through the boot camp of spiritual basics and build ourselves up in preparation for any higher calling and the further training that will entail. If we are consistent in our lifestyle of eating a healthy spiritual and physical diet and properly exercising spiritually and physically our way will become evident. We will discover where we are particularly gifted and where we are especially interested. We may never become one of the world's household names either spiritually or physically, but that's ok.

Whether you desire to be an endurance runner, a weight lifter or a weekend warrior; a prophesy guru or child's Sunday school teacher, there is more than one way to get Christ Fit. This is exactly why as a trainer I am steering well clear of professing to have the next big thing to help you achieve your fitness goals. I don't have a nickel in this quarter. If you are led to do Zumba, Insanity, pump iron, jog…? Go for it. Just pick something you will and can stick with and do it. If you want to go to a Baptist church, non-denominational, become a missionary; serve in your church's coffee bar…? Go for it. There is only "One Way," and that way is Jesus Christ, but there is more than one way to be Christ Fit. Eat a healthy spititual and physical diet. Exercise spiritually and physically. Do them both consistently.

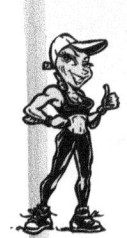

There is more than one way to get Christ Fit.
Let Jesus help you find your way.

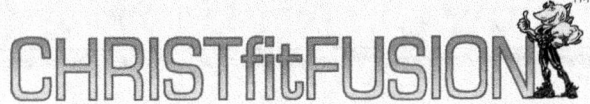

CHRISTfitFUSION™

Eat a Healthy Spiritual and Physical Diet. Exercise Spiritually and Physically. Do Them Both Consistently.

DATE:

SPIRITUAL DIET: PHYSICAL DIET:

SPIRITUAL EXERCISE: PHYSICAL EXERCISE:

NOTES:

Day 18 - *The Mirror Test*

Have you ever looked in the mirror and thought to yourself, "Self, we're getting out of shape!" It doesn't happen overnight though does it? You first start seeing little bulges and bits of flab in certain places. Stand naked in front of a mirror and jump up and down. When you stop jumping, whatever else doesn't is fat and that's what has to go. On the flip side of the coin; maybe you've had some muscle in the past and filled out places in your clothes (in a good way) that are now saggy and baggy. For guys we call that furniture disease (when your chest falls into your drawers).

You may look in the mirror and say, "I'm not 'that' out of shape. At least I'm not as fat as 'so and so.'" But could you improve? And why wouldn't you? Again, you're NOT striving for "perfection," but rather investing in your future and a quality of life that you just won't have otherwise.

Did you know that your body starts to deteriorate somewhere around your mid 20's. Unless you fight the natural progression of things you will start to lose lean muscle, your metabolism will slow down, you will grow warts, and your breath will stink (2 of the 4 are false. You figure it out). Now, you can still grow old without being fit. And yes, you are still going to get a little saggy no matter what. But, you can dramatically improve your quality of life by living a fitness lifestyle that you can start right now. Then by the time you're in your 80's you can carry your own groceries and tie your own shoes. Just imagine; you won't have to switch to Velcro laces or slip-ons. Woo Hoo!

Have you looked at your spiritual mirror lately; naked and vulnerable? Where are you starting to put on a few extra pounds spiritually? What spiritual muscles have started to atrophy due to lack of use? Even if you can say to yourself, "Self, at least we're not as sinful as 'that' person. At least we don't sin in 'that' way. We're not 'THAT' out of shape spiritually," do we ever get into "good enough" spiritual shape? Do we ever get "close enough" to God? If we're honest with ourselves we all have some spiritual fat to lose and some Godly muscle to gain.

And just like our physical bodies, we don't just find ourselves suddenly out of shape spiritually either. We get there by sliding a little bit at a time. We let spiritual junk food and influences into our lifestyle. Sometimes it's a substitute for something of more nutritional value. Ever catch yourself watching morning TV or a late night movie instead of reading your Bible, studying or reading a good book that will help you grow spiritually? Maybe our lifestyle gets crowded with things that keep us from getting in our spiritual workouts. It could be that we run out of time because we're too busy with work, baseball games or social events. It could even be that we volunteer so much of our time at church that we end up cutting our personal spiritual workout time with God short. There's nothing wrong with helping out at church if God has called you to it and as long as it isn't just "works" keeping you busy without the opportunity to grow.

Stand in front of your spiritual mirror and take a good look. Where do you need to drop a few pounds and tighten up? Where do you need to start working out to build those spiritual muscles back up? Don't get overwhelmed. You didn't get out of shape all at once and you're not going to get back in shape over-night either. Just start by committing to some simple spiritually healthy choices and get back on the road to becoming Christ Fit.

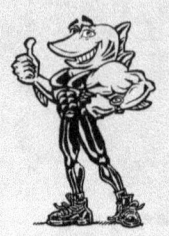

Looking intently into a mirror is intimidating, but it's honest. What is your spiritual and physical mirror showing you?

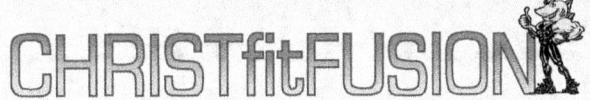

Eat a Healthy Spiritual and Physical Diet. Exercise Spiritually and Physically. Do Them Both Consistently.

DATE:

SPIRITUAL DIET: PHYSICAL DIET:

SPIRITUAL EXERCISE: PHYSICAL EXERCISE:

NOTES:

Compare a lack of a fitness lifestyle to not exercising your spiritual muscles. What happens; the same thing right? Atrophy and complaisance creep in. You can tell when you've been slacking off and if you've "let it go" for too long. It's way better to stay in shape than to have to get it back. And yes, God will always meet you where you are, no matter how far you've strayed. But just because he forgives you it doesn't mean you're not going to have to start working out again, do your spiritual exercises and go through some soreness and spiritual growing pains.

I remember a time that I was a little out of shape spiritually. Not totally out of shape; just starting to get a little soft and not quite as strong. I was still going to church "when I could", praying, and even reading my Bible relatively consistently. So I was working out spiritually (a little bit), but there were some components missing. I didn't have the complete "Lifestyle." I decided to get into a home Bible study group and broaden my spiritual exercise of fellowship, support and accountability. I needed to "up my game" a little bit so to speak. Well I'll be darn if I didn't land in a home group with what I thought were some of the un-coolest people in my church. I didn't even get in the cool group with all the popular folks. "Oh well. I'll suffer through it," I thought. Over time, and it wasn't that long either, the Holy Spirit showed me that I was right where God wanted me. I had been the goober all along and my home group was full of cool Christians that God had already planned to use in my life. I had totally been missing out on part of my spiritual lifestyle that was keeping me from being as spiritually fit as I could be and I didn't even know it. So now it's fixed and I'm back to being a Christian stud again. Wrong, but not giving up.

The point is the old cliché, "Use it or lose it." If you stop jogging or walking your cardiovascular endurance suffers because of it. Stop pumping iron and your muscles shrink. And no, muscles do not "turn into" fat. Muscle cells do not "turn into" fat cells. They are different cells altogether. Spiritual thoughts do not "turn into" sinful thoughts. Muscle cells shrink when unused and that slows down your metabolic rate therefore making it easier for fat cells to grow. Sinful thought's and deeds prevail when Godly ones are not exercised.

So what's it going to be? Are you going to use and strengthen your spiritual and physical muscles or are you going to let yourself become weak and unfit spiritually and physically? Fight the natural progression of a downward spiral. Eat a healthy spiritual and physical diet. Exercise and train spiritually and physically. Do them both consistently. Become and stay Christ Fit.

Seven days without spiritual and physical fitness makes one weak!

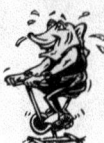

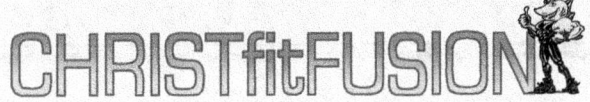

CHRISTfitFUSION™

Eat a Healthy Spiritual and Physical Diet. Exercise Spiritually and Physically. Do Them Both Consistently.

DATE:

SPIRITUAL DIET: PHYSICAL DIET:

SPIRITUAL EXERCISE: PHYSICAL EXERCISE:

NOTES:

Have you ever heard someone talk about how good of shape they "used to be in?" or How close they "used to be with the Lord." They were their "glory days" so to speak. What happened? Granted you're going to grow old no matter what and you are going to slow down a little. There is no fountain of youth, but what I want to drive home to you is this; Don't "let it go." Ever!

Look at the longevity of Billy Graham, Jerry Rice, Mother Teresa, and all the 80 year old marathon runners still out there. My papa was a WWII vet that lost half of both legs; one from the knee down and half of the other one length ways. It too was eventually cut off at the knee. He had been buried by logs in a log truck accident and lived; lost three children tragically (one was my dad); lost his wife and battled cancer for years. In his later years as he neared death whenever you'd ask him how he was doing he'd say "I have my good days and I have my better days." He never really had a bad day, just good and better and he always had a smile and an encouraging word.

My grandpa also served in WWII. He did not lose any limbs, but did have an equally difficult life in many ways and did also outlive his wife. When grandma died grandpa did too on the inside. He took up smoking to shorten his lifespan (which didn't work); became depressed and withdrawn and lost his health. He had once been a strong collegiate wrestler and football player. He even swam a mile every day after work during his senior years. But in the end he virtually pined himself to death.

Both men knew God and grandpa even did some preaching and taught Sunday school. I don't want to take away the significance of the grief grandpa must have felt when he lost his mate, but if all we have are our glory days then what good are we when we reach those golden years or get beyond our prime?

When I was in high school I participated in sports and was very competitive. What I lacked in stature I made up for with hustle, toughness and pure grit. I was a "late bloomer." On into college I finally caught my growth spurt and filled out when I really started hitting the weights and bodybuilding. I've kept in shape over the years and now looking back; many of the guys that used to out run and out lift me would have trouble out performing me at anything other than a belly flop contest.

It is fun to reminisce and talk about the glory days, but that can't be all we have. We've got to press on. Our work isn't done on this earth until we're taken out of it. There's still work to do and we'll be that much better equipped to do it when we're Christ Fit. So don't let yourself go; physically or spiritually. The good news is this; even if you do it's never too late. As long as you have breath in your lungs; it's never too late to draw a line in the sand and start making progress. You may never regain your prime, but you don't have to go down without a fight.

Start today if you haven't already. Eat a Healthy Spiritual and Physical Diet. Exercise Spiritually and Physically. Do Them Both Consistently. Do it for the rest of your life and you will live your glory days daily.

Glory days are fun to reminisce about but don't let it be all you have. There are still milestones ahead, achievements and memories to be made. Keep striving to be Christ Fit.

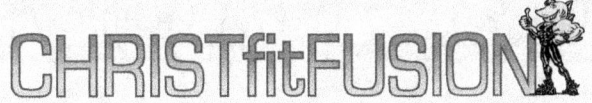

Eat a Healthy Spiritual and Physical Diet. Exercise Spiritually and Physically. Do Them Both Consistently.

DATE:

SPIRITUAL DIET: PHYSICAL DIET:

SPIRITUAL EXERCISE: PHYSICAL EXERCISE:

NOTES:

To be fit, really fit, takes an incredible amount of discipline and commitment. Think about the level of commitment that Olympic athletes make. Or consider professional athletes and their commitment to their teams and coaches and to themselves to be their best.

When I was bodybuilding during my college years my workout partner and I would train for two to three hours a day. I kept a training journal and documented every rep of every set of every exercise of every workout. I kept a journal for years and made very detailed notes about my development, successes and even failures. I kept a diet journal as well. I kept track of every calorie, gram of protein, carb, fat, water intake and sodium intake etc. You name it. Back then I could tell you how many calories and nutrients were in a ketchup packet. I was totally committed to my training and to being in the best shape that I could possibly be in. It was a lot of work and required extreme discipline. Sometimes it was even an inconvenience. But in the long run it was worth it and paid off because I won the first bodybuilding competition that I ever entered. It was what I had been training for. It was my goal and it was what I was committed to achieving. I was in the best shape of my life. I had trained for years. I had paid my dues. But my victory came with a price. There was no easy way or short cut. No magic bullet or magic workout routine. I trained for 1000's of hours, sweated my brains out, and strained every muscle fiber in my body to its max. I ate when I wasn't hungry, hit the gym instead of a movie, and pushed myself beyond limits.

What if we trained our spirit with that same tenacity? What if we disciplined ourselves like we were on an elite professional sports team? I mean think about it... Shouldn't we want to be on God's "A" team? I know that he doesn't show favoritism. And granted, a "c" string player is just as much a part of the team as an "a" string player, but c'mon... If we truly believe what we say we believe shouldn't we, wouldn't we, out of a hunger and thirst to be our best for the most awesome head coach ever, train ourselves like we had a purpose?

When we work out we have a goal don't we? And that goal is to stay in shape or get into better shape. Sure, we can enjoy the workout, but there is a goal. And the real fun is when our hard work pays off and we achieve our goals. Set a goal to get into the best spiritual shape of your life. Start training like you mean it. Don't be content with just sitting on the sidelines. Get Christ Fit and get in the game. But beware, as long as you're on the side lines the opposing team really doesn't treat you as a threat. But just like in a football game. Once you step out onto the playing field you're fair game to be hit (unless you're Tom Brady) so you had better be in shape.

Set your goals. Don't just go through the motions. Step up your training. Get in the word, listen to some radio teaching when you're in the car, serve your church family and neighbors, love God and people. Eat your Wheaties, put in the miles, and push yourself. Yes it takes commitment; serious commitment. But although God has a sense of humor he is a serious God that wants our best. Eat a healthy spiritual and physical diet, exercise properly spiritually and physically, and do them both consistently! The results will happen and you will be Christ Fit.

> **There's a difference between interest and commitment. When you're interested in doing something, you do it only when it's convenient. When you're committed to something, you accept no excuses; only results.**

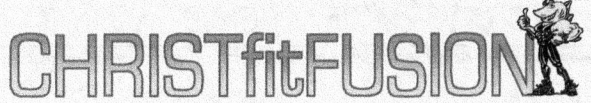

Eat a Healthy Spiritual and Physical Diet. Exercise Spiritually and Physically. Do Them Both Consistently.

DATE:

SPIRITUAL DIET: PHYSICAL DIET:

SPIRITUAL EXERCISE: PHYSICAL EXERCISE:

NOTES:

How many plans fail because there was no plan? How many plans fail because the plan was poor? How many plans fail because the plan was good, but the support system wasn't in place or adequate enough? How many plans just didn't have the right information to succeed in the first place?

I've had my failures. Some have been spiritual and some have been physical. With all of them there could have been some better planning. I've also succeeded at some things. Some have been spiritual and some have been physical. I can't think of anything that I succeeded at that I didn't plan for and work hard for.

So you become a Christian... That's new. What if you didn't necessarily plan to, but now that you are one you should probably make a plan. And honestly…the person that led you to Christ should make a plan too. What do I do with this person now that they "believed?"

If you are going to change your life in any way you should make a plan first. But how do you make a plan if you don't know what to do after the moment of your decision to change something.

Let's assume that you accept the Lord in a church or at a conference and you don't know anything about Christianity. Even better let's assume that somehow, supernaturally (imagine that…the Bible being supernatural…) you decide to follow Christ because He just touches you like He did Saul on the road to Damascus. The problem is that you don't really know what to do after establishing the fact that you believe. You have no plan.

When God got a hold of Saul and took control of his life Saul didn't have a plan. Well, actually he did; just not one that lined up with God. But when he encountered God he just knew his plans were changing.

Make your plans, but even if you already know Jesus, don't be afraid to have a Saul moment. Maybe your eyes need to get opened to a new plan. The same God that took Saul (the Saul with a plan) and made him into Paul the apostle (with "the" plan) can change your plans too. He took a Christian murdering thug and wrote most of the New Testament through him. Are you going to tell me that the same God can't tell you what and what not to eat… what and what not to do for exercise…? Are you going to tell me that he won't lead you to the right people to get you lined out like he did Saul with Ananias? Make your plans, but just know that your plans are subject to change and don't be so proud that you aren't willing to let God's plans become your plans when he intervenes in your life and puts people in it that need to lead you to truth.

When He does and when you know that He is guiding you then let Him lead you and let your plans be made to follow where He is leading you because then you will know that the plan, although full of trials, will not fail.

Whether spiritual or physical when making a plan your first step should be to go to God in prayer and talk to Him and listen to what He has to say. As you seek His guidance He will lead you. Plan now to obey.

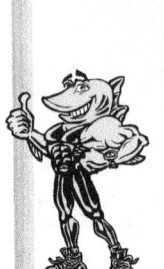

Proverbs 16:9: "We can make our plans, but the LORD determines our steps."

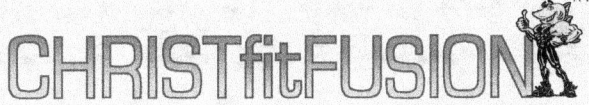

Eat a Healthy Spiritual and Physical Diet. Exercise Spiritually and Physically. Do Them Both Consistently.

DATE:

SPIRITUAL DIET: PHYSICAL DIET:

SPIRITUAL EXERCISE: PHYSICAL EXERCISE:

NOTES:

There are a lot of people in the gym that are doing things completely wrong and it is often very difficult to determine who they are. They look pretty good physically, but they are doing their exercises totally incorrectly. They are muscular and/or lean and look better than most, but the way they are performing their exercises is not going to get them to their goal. Or is it? I guess it depends on their goal.

They are in the gym for hours, they sweat like hookers in a jalapeño patch, they lift more pounds than a circus elephant, and they seem like they have a mission. But do they? The way they work out you'd think that they were in training for a serious competition, but most of the time they are just trying to look better than the person working out across from them. There is a TREMENDOUS difference between "working out" and "training."

Most of the people who "workout" desire to look better than most of the people around them so that they can brag about and feel good about their personal achievements and how much better in shape they are... Those that "train" know that they may not lift as many pounds or look as impressive during the training, but their end goal is to win a prize that can only be given to those that are disciplined and committed to doing things the right way and to the very end. Even if your goal is a personal one you need to "train" for it and not simply "workout."

If you've ever been in a gym then you've seen the "lat pull down." It is supposed to simulate the chin up, but most of the time it looks like the person doing the exercise is rowing a boat up a wall. Almost every exercise gets cheated on for the sake of looking good and strong for others within eyeshot.

Most of the beasts in the gym and most of the beauties have never competed in a contest. They can afford to cheat because they can still look better than most but never have to put their muscle where their mouth is.

Those that compete and win the prize "train" for it. They don't just "workout." They do exercises the right way even if it doesn't look as impressive to on lookers. They don't overload themselves in an attempt to impress someone in the short term. They focus on the true training that will get them to the prize they desire. The reason they win the prize is because they are disciplined enough to do the exercises the right way in order to develop their bodies in such a way that only a true judge with an expert eye will appreciate.

Be careful who you follow. Don't base everything on impressiveness. Don't be fooled by someone who just looks the part. Get with someone who has a track record. Follow those that practice what they preach. Follow people of character and discipline who will help you train and not just break a sweat.

If you want to become Christ Fit then get discipled. Get trained. Get mentored. Don't just follow the teachings of someone wanting to appear "Christian." It is hard to tell sometimes though. Just like it's hard to tell who is working out vs. training in the gym. There is nothing wrong with getting some help and some guidance. Just seek out the person most interested in helping you and pointing you to Jesus rather than impressing you with what they can do or have done.

Just because everyone else is doing it doesn't mean everyone else is doing it right.

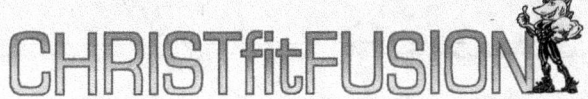

CHRISTfitFUSION™

Eat a Healthy Spiritual and Physical Diet. Exercise Spiritually and Physically. Do Them Both Consistently.

DATE:

SPIRITUAL DIET: PHYSICAL DIET:

SPIRITUAL EXERCISE: PHYSICAL EXERCISE:

NOTES:

Working out may feel awkward at first. Stick with it. It'll become more natural.

Have you ever tried praying for the first time in a long time or maybe for the first few times ever? Remember how it felt awkward; especially praying "out loud?" Stick with it. It'll become natural. You'll get it. So consider this with exercise. Whether it's for the first time or the first time in a long time you should start slow enough that you allow your body to get stronger and grow healthier without damaging it along the way by trying to achieve things you're not capable of. Think about it. You don't make a decision to get into shape and then immediately go out and attempt to climb Mt. Everest. Just start slow, build up, and eventually, with consistency, you'll be running bleachers, jumping cars, and winning funny painful Japanese game shows.

When you first do an aerobics class or Zumba etc., the steps are awkward. When you press a weight over your head for the first time or the first time in a long time there is some unsteadiness. When you first do those aerobics steps or weights you have the ability you just don't have the rhythm, coordination or stability. It takes more than being able to put one foot in front of the other to do Zumba. You have to develop the necessary coordination and rhythm. The reason you feel unsteady when you first press a weight over your head is because although you have the muscle strength to do it there are intricate stabilizing muscles around your joints that are undeveloped and have to get stronger in order for you to be able to lift the weights without wobbling. That's one reason why you want to start off slow and build up to more strenuous exercises. If you don't you can easily injure the more delicate stabilizers and ground yourself before you ever even take off.

So start slow, be consistent and stay with it. I'm not telling you to avoid breaking a sweat or to avoid pushing yourself. Just be careful and don't over work / over train yourself before you're ready. Whether starting strength training or aerobic activity use lighter weights and less intensity until things become more natural and stable.

Don't be anymore discouraged if some things feel awkward spiritually. It's normal and has happened to everyone at some point. Whether a new Christian or just getting back into the spiritual gym, things are just going to feel awkward at first. It can feel really strange to pray when you're not used to it. It can feel strange to pray out loud with your family at a restaurant. Heck, it can feel awkward to pray with your family at home if you've never done it. It feels strange to sit in someone's living room with people you don't know very well and do a small group Bible study. It can feel especially awkward to open up and share in that environment or even privately with a close friend. But don't give up. Stick with it and be consistent. Take it slow at first and don't try to lift the whole gym. As you get stronger and more trained up; as your spiritual stabilizing muscles get stronger and more developed things will become a lot more natural and you'll be able to do these spiritual exercises easily and well on your way to being Christ Fit.

So for now just stay consistent, be diligent, start slow if you need to and progress as you can. It's not like you're being asked to compete in a sport or teach an aerobics class. It's not like you're expected to share your faith on stage or lead a home Bible study. Not yet anyway. The thing about getting Christ Fit though is that you're never done. You're always improving and as you get in better shape you'll find that you have to challenge yourself with things that give you those awkward feelings all over again. It's part of the process.

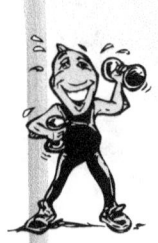

**Inches make miles. Seconds make hours.
Pounds make tons.**

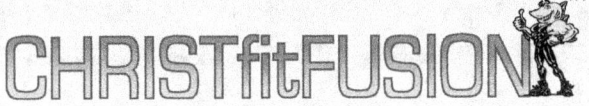

DATE:

SPIRITUAL DIET: PHYSICAL DIET:

SPIRITUAL EXERCISE: PHYSICAL EXERCISE:

NOTES:

When I was a little boy I had an uncle named Freddie. Freddie was not in particularly great shape, but he could pop his pecs (flex his chest muscles individually and make his man boobs dance). It was sooo cool and I had to be able to do it. Later it was Hulk Hogan and Sylvester Stallone that caught my attention and they had the total package to go along with the bouncing bulges of sex appeal.

Years later after countless hours in the gym I achieved my goal of the peck popping (I know, TMI). I even competed in and won a state bodybuilding competition. However, I just never could get my chest as thick and round looking as the other Brutus Beefcakes. My bounces were just not as impressive. I was in great shape, but I wasn't content. I wanted what the other guys had. I wanted "their" pecs. The trouble with that desire was the fact that I just didn't have the genetics to build those kinds of muscles. I could make what I had bigger and stronger, but I was limited in the way my muscles were shaped and in my ability for obtaining a body builder's physique. My genetics were actually predisposed for endurance running and cross training type sports.

Enough about me; the point I want to make with the story is that we've all been given a shape and a genetic propensity. We can improve upon that shape and even a 98 lb. weakling can grow some muscles. Even a defensive lineman for the Dallas Cowboys can get in shape to run a 10K. Neither will be as good as the other because of the way they are made. The 98 lb. weakling will run circles around the big guy and the big guy will use the 98 lb. weakling as a warm up set in the gym. It's fine to do whatever you want to do as physical exercise, just realize that not everyone is going to look like a movie star.

Another point is that there truly are genetically gifted freaks of nature. Some people can get away with murder when it comes to diet and exercise. Some do get amazing results compared to the efforts they put in.

Don't covet your neighbor's pecs. Learn to have realistic goals and expectations. "The secret to a dancers body" is not a dance video or special diet. The secret is genetics, dancing your butt off for hours and sometimes not eating as much as you want. Focus on your personal progress, not perfection. And remember, fitness is more than what you look like on the outside. Jesus called the Pharisees white washed tombs because they had spiritual six pack abs and could pop their religious pecs, but their cholesterol was over 400.

We all have spiritual predisposition. We all have our gifts and were specifically designed by God. We can't all be spiritual weight lifters. Just because someone has the gift of preaching or tongues or whatever else doesn't make them any more spiritually fit than anyone else. The truth is it's best for us all to do a little cross training both spiritually and physically. Runners should lift a little weight. Weight lifters should do a little cardio. But when it comes to our God given shape, design, gift, purpose and spiritual genetics we can only maximize on what we've already been blessed with.

Don't covet your neighbor's pecs. Maximize the talent God has given you and no matter what that is, you will become Christ Fit. Eat a Healthy Spiritual and Physical Diet. Exercise Spiritually and Physically. Do Them Both Consistently. Simple. Challenging. Effective. Live the right lifestyle and let the results take care of themselves.

**You can only make what you already have better.
You are you and there is nothing wrong with that.**

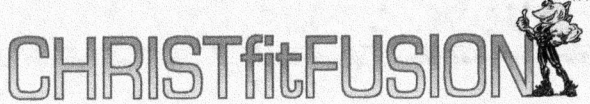

Eat a Healthy Spiritual and Physical Diet. Exercise Spiritually and Physically. Do Them Both Consistently.

DATE:

SPIRITUAL DIET: PHYSICAL DIET:

SPIRITUAL EXERCISE: PHYSICAL EXERCISE:

NOTES:

Yes, you should take it slow in the beginning. But, even then you need to be tenacious. Whether you're trying to get some of the basic fundamental truths about living a Christian lifestyle or studying end times prophesy you need to be tenacious. Even when just starting out we should have a vigor and enthusiasm in our spiritual journey. It's the same with our physical exercise. Even if you're out of shape and starting from scratch you can still have a tenacious attitude with what little bit you can handle. Don't just go through the motions. Put some energy into it and take breaks when you need them.

It's kind of like swatting flies, which if you're at my house is like an Olympic sport. When you go to swat a fly you don't just casually fling the fly swatter in the fly's general direction. Heck no! You swat deliberately at that little sucker with a purpose. And if you miss! "Oh, it's on now!" You'll swat again and again and again. You'll be waving that fly swatter like it's a Jedi light saver. Shoot, you'll even take shots at him while he's flying or landing on the ceiling fan. "TENACIOUS!" Now that's a work out right there.

Starting out slow and combining that with tenaciousness can seem contradictory. But what about this; what if instead of lifting so much weight that you strain something and get too sore to do it again for a week, you lift a light weight that is almost embarrassingly handled for 20-30 repetitions. Do that over and over again for a few weeks, but do it with an energy level of swatting a fly. What if instead of getting into an aerobics class of some kind right off the bat you step up and down the first step of your house 100 times in a row for a couple of weeks? Whether you're pressing 45 pounds 20 times on the bench press or stepping up and down 1 step in your house; that's starting slow and you can be tenacious doing it.

You don't have to just go through the motions. It's low impact enough that you can really get after it, be effective, feel and know that you've accomplished something and still be ready to do it again the next day and also know when it's time to challenge yourself with the next level.

So how can we be tenacious in our spiritual fitness? What does that mean exactly? It means this. Whether you're reading the gospel of John (a book widely recommended to new believers) for the first time or charting into new territory as a seasoned believer, don't bite off more than you can chew, but what you can chew; chew with a veracity of a duck getting after a June bug.

Be tenacious. You're not going to get far without it. Whether you're trying to improve fitness spiritually or physically, simply going through the motions is ineffective. I've seen many a person get on a tread mill day after day and walk 100's of miles over the course of several months and not lose a single pound. No doubt there are other issues in play as well and if they're as enthusiastic about their diet and overall lifestyle as they are about their time on the tread mill it's a wonder they ever even get out of bed. On the other hand I've seen people get on the tread mill and bust out a 15-20 minute cardio session, pound out a 15-20 minute weight workout and be out the door before "Sleepy" ever gets warmed up. They spend less time, they're more tenacious, but they get twice the results.

You can read your Bible for hours and sit through countless sermons and there's nothing wrong with that, but you'll be wasting your time if you're just going through the motions. Be deliberate, be tenacious, do what you can handle and add to your repertoire when you're ready for it.

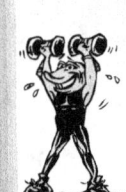

Whether you're swatting flies or climbing stairs at the mall... be tenacious.

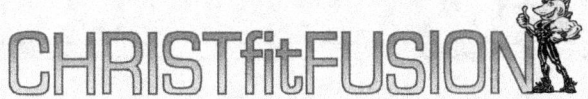

Eat a Healthy Spiritual and Physical Diet. Exercise Spiritually and Physically. Do Them Both Consistently.

DATE:

SPIRITUAL DIET: PHYSICAL DIET:

SPIRITUAL EXERCISE: PHYSICAL EXERCISE:

NOTES:

Yep, it's true, and yes, take it slow in the beginning and strengthen those stabilizing muscles first. Yes, gradually build up to more challenging workouts. But don't think for a minute that spiritual and physical fitness isn't going to involve some pain because it is. The good news is that sometimes it's a good pain.

When we grow there is some pain involved along the way. Whether physical or spiritual there are growing pains. Since day one as children we experienced growing pains in our legs and other extremities as we grew.

Barbells stress our muscles and make them burn. Walking, hiking and running make our legs burn. They are stresses that challenge our bodies and with the right diet in place our bodies adapt to that stress in order to get stronger. We also have spiritual challenges and stressors that cause us to grow spiritually if we have the right spiritual diet in place. Sometimes it hurts. Ok a lot of the time it hurts, but we get stronger if we stay with the program and stick to the Christ Fit lifestyle. Eat a healthy spiritual and physical diet, exercise and train spiritually and physically and do them both consistently.

If there isn't some pain, some stretching your limits, some burning and pushing through it then you're probably not challenging yourself enough. Not every workout has to be a crippling, exhausting event that leaves you on the floor in a puddle of sweat. If they do then you're overtraining and will likely burn out, plateau or injure yourself eventually. But there does need to be some sweat equity involved and some strain in the process.

When we exercise it's a challenge. Or at least it should be. Whether pumping iron, walking/jogging, or playing a sport we need to "feel the burn" so to speak. When we get into better shape we can handle some of those punishing workouts where we feel like we can't move a muscle when we're done.

Whether it's a workout early on in your fitness career or a drop dead bone crusher after you've become fit enough to handle it, that burn and that pain you endure is actually doing trauma to your body and its muscles. But the human body is amazing. It learns how to adapt to that stress so that it is less traumatizing and can better cope with it. It gets stronger and develops more lung capacity and endurance. Think about the last time you got a blister from raking leaves or doing something else with your hands that you aren't used to doing. That blister is a result of trauma. But, if you work with your hands every day your hands will adapt to that stress and cope with it by developing calluses. No more blisters. Until that is, you do something above and beyond your normal leaf raking that causes your hands to be traumatized again. More blisters…Unless of course you maintain that extra stress repeatedly over time and give your hands additional stress that they have to adapt to.

That's essentially what happens with your muscles. Workout once every so often and all you get is "blisters" every time. Do it regularly and you adapt to it. The caveat is that your muscles need proper nutrition in order to adapt to the stress. Without proper protein, carbs, and fats your muscles just aren't going to be able to recover and adapt.

So let's talk spiritual exercise for a minute. Hopefully you've had the chance to experience the pain of a spiritual blister. Maybe it was a convicting Easter sermon or a message you heard at a religious conference or Bible study that you took action on, but never stuck with. Whatever the case I hope you've strained your spiritual muscles and felt the exhilaration of going through the exercise and feeling the pain of the blister later.

Whenever we decide to act on what God is telling us to do it's going to cause us to strain our spiritual muscles. Even when it is too much for us to handle He is there to spot us. It's going to be uncomfortable during the exercise and there's going to be some soreness after. If we stay with it instead of running away from the pain we'll be getting Christ Fit. It won't be long before the little spiritual exercise He first gave us is a breeze. It'll seem like a light weight. It also won't be long before it's time to handle a tougher exercise routine. And it's that never ending journey of getting into a little better shape and then pushing ourselves to that next level again and again that keeps us on the road to becoming Christ Fit.

Work through the pain. It won't be long before 1 mile isn't enough. 1 chapter isn't enough. 10 lbs. isn't enough. Church once a week isn't enough. You'll need and want more.

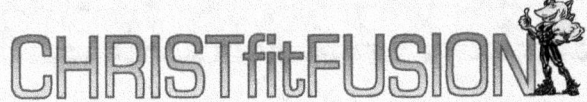

CHRISTfitFUSION™

Eat a Healthy Spiritual and Physical Diet. Exercise Spiritually and Physically. Do Them Both Consistently.

DATE:

SPIRITUAL DIET: PHYSICAL DIET:

SPIRITUAL EXERCISE: PHYSICAL EXERCISE:

NOTES:

This battle seems to have been going on since before the Dead Sea was even sick. "Do cardio if you want to lose weight," "Pump iron if you want to bulk up." "Do cardio if you want a healthy cardio vascular system," "Pump iron if you want to get strong." Ladies typically don't want to "bulk up," they just want to be lean so they don't want to do strength training very seriously.

I'm going to get on my soap box on this one and line this out for you. First of all, the best looking bodies on the planet spend time doing resistance training of some kind. They "pump iron." There, I said it. What I didn't say is that they avoid cardio at all cost. But what if they did? What about the beasts that stand on stage and flex their giant muscles? I'm not going to make the case that they have the best looking bodies or the healthiest, especially those that abuse steroids etc. That's very unbalanced and unhealthy on a whole different level. But there are some amazingly muscular freaks of nature out there that don't do steroids and also don't do hardly a lick of cardio. So they look good, fit, built and very lean with six pack abs, but their cardio vascular system is unhealthy, right? Nope, wrong. Although resistance training isn't necessarily aerobic (it's anaerobic) when you're fit enough to do it with enough intensity you can really elevate your heart rate and get extremely winded throughout the workout as well. But even that is beside the point. The goal of resistance training is to increase strength and or muscle size. What do muscles need? They need oxygen from the blood they get. The more developed the skeletal muscles get the more fit and efficient cardiac muscles have to become to supply the skeletal muscles with blood and oxygen. A "buff" person doing minimal cardio can have a heart rate just as low, can pump just as much blood and can uptake just as much oxygen as some runners.

So if someone who gravitates towards weights can have a healthy cardio vascular system; can a person who gravitates towards cardio have developed muscles? Have you ever observed a cyclist's or a speed skater's legs? Holy cow! So a 300 lb. NFL lineman can run around on a football field for 60 minutes. He's fit in his own right. A cardio athlete can have a muscular looking body. He's fit in his own right. So which is better, cardio or pumping iron? The simple answer is both. Especially for the lay person starting off on a Christ Fit journey. Take the well rounded approach and as you become fit if you want to focus on one more than the other then go for it. The fact of the matter is you need a balance of both. That's one reason why I combine the two when I teach a Christ Fit circuit training class. A circuit class is cardiovascular in nature because you don't stop moving. You go from one station to the next with no rest and the stations involve aerobic as well as resistance exercises.

Ladies, unless you are blessed (or cursed if you choose to look at it like that) with abnormally "Marvel Comic" testosterone you're not going to bulk up from staring at a weight too long. When your clothes feel a little tighter don't freak out. You're muscles have grown a little bit but more muscle increases your 24 hour calorie burn. Give the muscle a chance. In a little time you'll shrink your fat cells and your body will in turn shrink. Then you have nice lean muscle to show for it and your clothes will be too loose, giving you an excuse to go shopping.

What about spiritual fitness? If Jesus is in it then it's all good. Too much spirit and not enough Word can be unbalanced. Too much knowledge without enough application is useless. Getting hung up on which denomination or version of the Bible is wasting your time. Stop buying into myths. Educate yourself, study, workout your salvation with fear and trembling, but for goodness sake stop judging others and get busy on your own Christ Fit journey.

When comparing apples and oranges don't forget that they are both fruit.

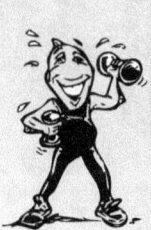

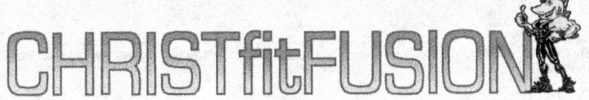

Eat a Healthy Spiritual and Physical Diet. Exercise Spiritually and Physically. Do Them Both Consistently.

DATE:

SPIRITUAL DIET: PHYSICAL DIET:

SPIRITUAL EXERCISE: PHYSICAL EXERCISE:

NOTES:

There's a cartoon drawing that I have loved for years. It's a picture of a crane (the bird) who is attempting to eat a frog head first. Apparently he has stooped down and grabbed the little guy by the head and stood up with him to finish the job, but the frog even with his head in the giant bird's beak and facing certain doom has the presence of mind to get his little hands wrapped around the bird's throat to prevent him from swallowing. The caption says, "Never Ever Give Up!" There's another quote that I like. I don't know where it came from, but my dad used to say all the time, "When you get to the end of your rope, tie a knot and hang on." Have you ever felt like the frog or felt like you were about to slip off the end of your rope? I have. Never ever give up.

I've already addressed issues like keeping your Christ Fit lifestyle sustainable so you don't burn out, having balance, focusing on progress rather than perfection etc. But sometimes no matter what all you do right you still find yourself in a situation that requires pure grit and determination. Never just let yourself go, even when you have a dry spell or a setback. Even when circumstances keep you from living the Christ Fit lifestyle like you want to. Don't give up and don't let yourself go. Keep some sort of momentum going even if it's not as much as you'd like. I know it's tempting at times. I know when you're discouraged it's easy to think "Oh, what's the use?" Stop it. Capture every thought, keep your eyes on Jesus and never ever give up.

It really stinks to make progress, get results, and then have to start all over again from scratch. You work so hard, endure the pain and hardships and then have to do it all over again. Don't ever let yourself go. Whatever it takes; even if you can only squeeze in a 10 minute workout, do it. Whatever it takes you keep pushing. Grab that bird by the throat and don't let him swallow you.

From time to time it's going to happen. You're going to miss a day and not read your Bible. You're going to miss church. You're going to go back to a bad habit. You're going to get down on yourself for being weak and going back to that web site or for giving in to the fast food. And the more you slip the easier it is to keep slipping and eventually give in and say, "What's the use? I quit. I can't do it. It's too hard." Tighten your grip and don't give up. You can do it. You can press on. Use the resources God has given you. Stand on his promises and his truths. Lean on your workout / accountability partner. Do whatever it is you have to do.

But what if it's too late? What if you've already given up and let yourself go? What if you're in a spot where you do have to start from scratch? The good news is that God is faithful to forgive and restore you if you repent in your heart. Repenting is a change of heart. A turning away from sin and turning to God. So whether that means stopping something that you shouldn't be doing or starting something that you should be doing, repent and get on track. Repent daily or hourly if necessary, but whatever you do Never ever give up on becoming Christ Fit.

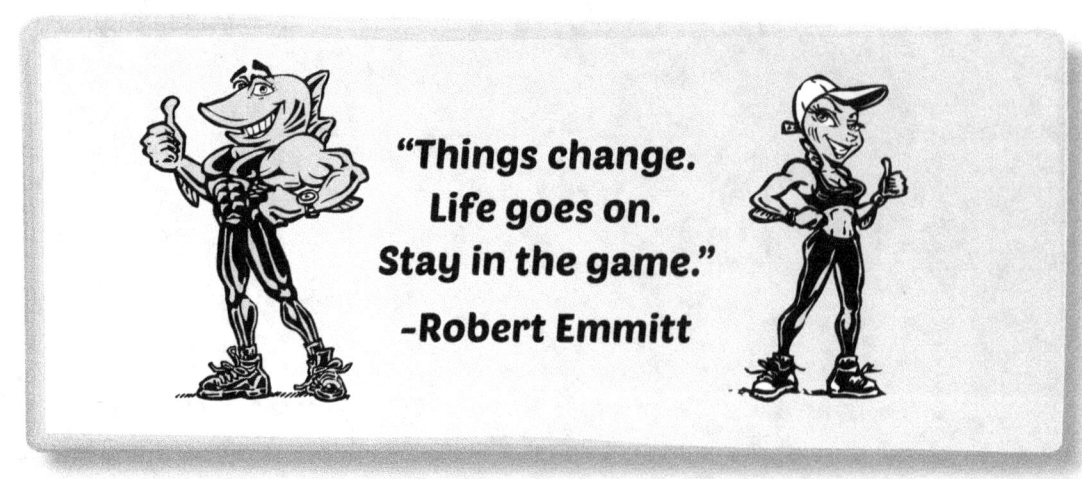

"Things change.
Life goes on.
Stay in the game."
-Robert Emmitt

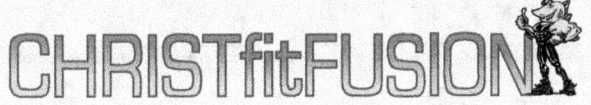

CHRISTfitFUSION™

Eat a Healthy Spiritual and Physical Diet. Exercise Spiritually and Physically. Do Them Both Consistently.

DATE:

SPIRITUAL DIET: PHYSICAL DIET:

SPIRITUAL EXERCISE: PHYSICAL EXERCISE:

NOTES:

Yes, we are in a fight. The Bible is clear that there is a spiritual battle being waged all around us at all times. There are moments when I think that I can literally feel it. As always, God is good. He has given us spiritual armor. The thing about armor is that it's heavy so you have to be fit to wear it. For those of you who have never been in an actual fight it's grueling and exhausting. A fight doesn't end until you either win, your opponent wins or someone else steps in and breaks it up.

The fight we're in has been thrust upon us. We weren't looking for it. We didn't ask for it, but we're smack dab in the middle of it whether we want to be or not. We have to "leave it in the ring." That's just a boxing expression for "give it all you've got." You're in the fight of your life and a mediocre effort isn't going to get the job done.

When I was in my mid 20's I entered a "Tough Man" boxing tournament. I didn't have any formal training in boxing, but I was pretty tough and I was very fit. I only fought one fight in the entire tournament. The matches were 3, 1 minute rounds. That's not much time, but let me tell you, it was truly fast and furious and a nonstop 110% effort. I don't remember how I made it out to the hotel's hallway outside the arena after the fight was over because I was so spent, but I did. And once there I lay down on the floor and didn't move for probably 30 minutes. I had left everything I had back there in the ring and had nothing left.

I had nothing left, but win lose or draw I also had no regrets. I had done everything that I possibly could to win. I couldn't have tried harder. I couldn't have landed more punches. I couldn't have done anything more than what I had done and I was satisfied with giving it my all.

Leave it in the ring people. Give it all you've got. At the end of your fight you don't want to look back and have regrets or wonder if you could've done just a little better if only you had… You don't want to look back and say I would have… or would have liked to… serve more, love more, known Jesus better, gone on those youth group trips, been a better parent, been a better steward so I could give more and help those in need, fill in the blank…

I know that to some degree we all have some regrets. There's no way that we are going to fight the perfect fight day in and day out like we should. But at the end of it all wouldn't it be great to look back and know that you fought hard and left it in the ring?

It's a long fight; a lot longer than 3, 1 minute rounds. The only way to survive is to train and be Christ Fit. Whether you're fighting a weight/health battle or a spiritual battle you have to get Christ Fit to fight it successfully. And yes, even food can be part of your spiritual battle. Anything can. Our opponent doesn't fight fair. He will hit you however and wherever he has to in order to take you down.

Take the fight seriously. Start training right now if you haven't already. Eat a healthy spiritual and physical diet. Exercise and train spiritually and physically. Do them both consistently. Take the fight head on and leave it in the ring. Fight in such a way that win, lose or draw, when the last bell rings you can know you did your best and have no regrets.

> **"It's not the will to win that matters. Everyone has that. It's the will to prepare to win that matters."**
>
> **-Paul "Bear" Bryant**

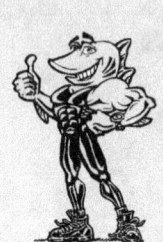

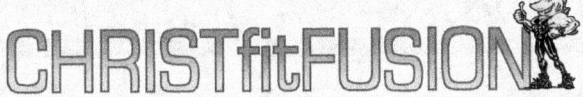

Eat a Healthy Spiritual and Physical Diet. Exercise Spiritually and Physically. Do Them Both Consistently.

DATE:

SPIRITUAL DIET: PHYSICAL DIET:

SPIRITUAL EXERCISE: PHYSICAL EXERCISE:

NOTES:

There's no way to recap this entire journal on one page. I hope you read it again and again. You'll most likely have to if you're on a mission to become Christ Fit. This is only a simple journal, but God truly inspired me to write it for whatever reason. I hope it has inspired you in some ways. Just like the "supplements" page, this journal is simply a supplement and a tool.

Do you ever get spiritual enough? Do you ever get fit enough? Heck no. So even if you've read the Bible from cover to cover and led Bible studies and gone on mission trips do you ever say to yourself, "Ok, I'm close enough to God now; I don't need to read my Bible anymore." If you do you can expect a tap on the shoulder from the Holy Spirit or maybe even a kick in the butt. We can never quit. We've got to keep training. The same goes for our fitness. We can never stop. We've got to keep fighting.

Our enemy never stops attacking us, never stops accusing and never throws in the towel. We're going to get hit. We're never strong enough, fit enough or tough enough to take him on. Don't ever get cocky and think you are. In the boxing tournament I mentioned previously I was in the best physical shape of my life. I was matched up with a tall skinny kid. I had this. Before the match started, remember that peck popping thing? Yup, I was doing that. I was a police officer at the time and I was about to put the "cuff and stuff" on this kid. Half way through the first round he broke my nose and I went down like a lead balloon. The few thousand in attendance roared and my 10 or so friends sitting ring side gasped. It was quite the humbling experience. I managed to get up by the count of 8 and was allowed to continue. Come to find out later, this kid had some boxing experience. Who knew? I spent the last half of that round covering up and running for my life. Folks, in our spiritual battles we're going to get hit and knocked down from time to time. Down, but not out. We can win the fight without winning every round. If we're Christ Fit enough we can survive until the bell rings and then get a breather. When the bell rang for me, ending the first round, I made it to my corner. I had a man from church as my corner man and he gave me some advice. Well, first of all he told me I couldn't win. "Gee, thanks." My opponent was too skilled and was going to kill me if I tried to go toe to toe and box with him. I was going to get hit and my corner man knew it. He gave me some advice to put myself in a position to at least be able to land some blows. People, the devil and his army are too powerful and too skilled for us to defeat. We have to listen to our corner man, the Holy Spirit, and follow his advice. I spent the last 2 rounds with my head buried into my opponent's chest. Pushing against him I was able to keep him on the ropes and although he was able to hit me he couldn't get a hard lick on me like he did before. At the same time I was able to pound away at his rib cage. I must have hit him 200 or 300 times in those last 2 minutes and as the last round was about to end I stepped back and came straight in with a hard right to his face, sending him back. He might have gone down, but he grabbed the ropes and stayed on his feet. The referee gave him a standing 8 count as the last bell rang. They ended up calling the match a draw. Never ever give up. For me it was a personal victory just to finish that fight. The following night I watched my opponent take second place overall and even though I didn't compete the second night because of my nose I had no regrets because I had done my best (I still secretly wonder sometimes though).

When we win a round or in some case win a personal spiritual fight, it's fun to celebrate and give praise. It's fine to take some time to recover. You just can't quit or take too much time off. The next fight, in some form or fashion, is already on the way and the opponents only get tougher as you get more Christ Fit, but you can do it.

Eat a healthy spiritual and physical diet. Exercise and train spiritually and physically. Do them both consistently. Don't believe the lies. If you want to know the secret to a dancer's body then enroll at Juilliard. If you want to burn 3 times the calories, do 3 times the exercise. The machine that combines the tread mill, stair climber, and elliptical doesn't do it (I used to assemble them. They're junk). There is no miracle drug, supplement, diet, machine or workout.

The only miracle is that Jesus died for our sins and gave us the opportunity to live forever through faith in him. He gave you one body. Take care of it; not only for your sake, but others as well.

Get accountability. Get a workout partner. Focus on progress rather than perfection, but definitely make progress. Start slow and build up. Don't overdo it, but certainly challenge yourself to reach new goals. Capture every thought and make wise choices. Look into your spiritual mirror as well as your physical one. Make the necessary adjustments when you need to. Make a plan. Be committed. Be tenacious. Get wise counsel from a trustworthy and reputable source. Educate and study for yourself so you will know the truth. Get on fire. Get excited and fire up your spiritual and physical metabolism. When you get knocked down, get back up. When you fail, stray, blow your diet or get off track, repent. Draw a line in the sand and press ahead. It's as simple as all of that.

Seriously, don't be overwhelmed. It really is simple. And it's a process. Live the right lifestyle and the results will take care of themselves. Eat a healthy spiritual and physical diet. Exercise and train spiritually and physically. Do them both consistently and you will be Christ Fit.

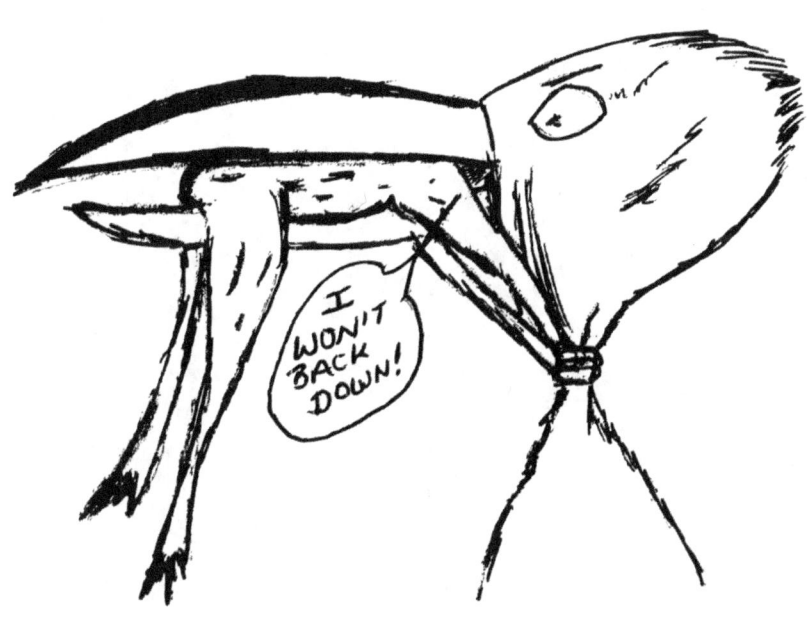

What is your fight? Food? Something else?
We all have one. We must get Christ Fit to do battle.
You've just made a great start.
Keep it up. Don't quit!

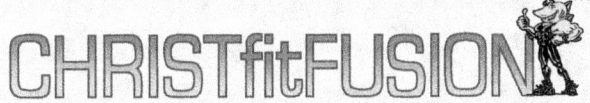

CHRISTfitFUSION

Eat a Healthy Spiritual and Physical Diet. Exercise Spiritually and Physically. Do Them Both Consistently.

DATE:

SPIRITUAL DIET: PHYSICAL DIET:

SPIRITUAL EXERCISE: PHYSICAL EXERCISE:

NOTES:

Rusty was raised in Searcy, Arkansas and is the oldest of three.

At an early age Rusty recognized his competitive spirit and always challenged himself mentally and physically. By the time he was 14 he was already the fastest back stroke swimmer in the state!

Being raised mostly by his grandparents, Rusty understood the effects of war as both his grandfathers served in the military. Living under that type of authority instilled a standard of serving of which only the military combined with a Christian environment is capable.

At 17 he enlisted with the National Guard as an Infantryman. He served for six years while also attending Harding University. After graduation, it wasn't long before he was accepted into the Little Rock, AR police academy where he graduated second in his class.

It was during this time in his life Rusty discovered fitness as a true passion. He began training to become a body builder. Once again he succeeded and won first place in his weight class as novice and fourth in the open class a couple years later.

People working out in the gym started asking him about his training and offered to pay for his assistance in their own training. Thus began the fitness training journey.

Rusty moved from Arkansas to California and while there certified as a personal fitness trainer through I.S.S.A. (International Sports Sciences Association) and operated his own mobile fitness business called Fitness to You.

He was highly successful and trained clients of all ages, all walks of life, and all having varying fitness challenges. Even though Rusty grew up going to church, it wasn't until this time in his life that he had his divine encounter with Jesus and became His follower. He attributed the success of his business to his walk with The Lord.

After years training clients off and on in various roles, Rusty came to the realization that the "clipboard" approach didn't seem to help anyone move towards the lifestyle change he knew they desperately needed. Only The Lord could make that type of dramatic change.

It was out of his desire to truly help people find The Lord and get fit that Christ Fit Fusion was birthed.

Currently Rusty lives with his wife Amy Jo, his two sons, Dillon and Cameron and his two step children Austin and Grace in San Antonio, TX.